Embrace the On-going Transformational Power of Spirit

There are few books that give you a direct, first-hand experience of truth—one that will stimulate your mind, open your heart, and feed your soul. *The Ultimate Cure* is such a book.

Dr. Jim Dreaver addresses the conflicts we all struggle with at times: physical health, emotional pain, relationships, money, and meaning and direction in work and life. He shows you how, through learning to be more present in the moment, you can heal these conflicts and awaken to an ever deeper source of love and joy within.

The book is about getting to know yourself as a multi-dimensional, spiritually alive human being. It is about undertaking a healing journey, one that will bring you to the intuitive realization that you are more than your body, mind, and circumstances—that your real nature is of Spirit. Once you have awakened to this, you will have access to an inexhaustible source of well-being, clarity, and inner freedom that no one can ever take from you. On your journey you will discover:

The limits of intellectual understanding

Breath as the key to life and health

The importance of being in your body

The yoga of awareness and feeling

The best diet for you

You are not your thoughts

Meditation: returning to your natural state of ease

The power of the present

Self-acceptance: the first enlightenment

How to heal the wounds of the past

The secret of dealing with problems

Crisis as a wake-up call

Work as a spiritual exercise

How the ego gets in the way

The lesson of non-attachment

The dance of Grace and will

The energy of Spirit is the source of everything you have been looking for. It is the energy of your aliveness. It is the well-spring of your creativity. It is your passion. It is your joy. It is your ability to think, to dream, to laugh, to feel. It is your essence. It is the love you have longed for all your life. It is who and what you are. It really is the ultimate cure for whatever is ailing you.

About the Author

Dr. Jim Dreaver has been leading workshops on healing and transformation since 1978. A native of New Zealand, he served as an artillery officer in Vietnam during the Tet offensive. Later he became one of the youngest captains in the New Zealand army, before leaving the military to work in sales for two years. He graduated with honors from Palmer College of Chiropractic in 1976.

In 1975, at the age of 29, Dr. Dreaver went through a life-threatening health crisis which started him down the self-realization path. His quest has taken him to yoga ashrams in India, and to Buddhist temples in the Himalayas of Nepal. His studies of various spiritual teachings, including those of the renowned J. Krishnamurti, have given him many of the insights contained in this book. His work focuses on combining both Eastern and Western approaches to transformation, along with the lessons of his own life experience, and presenting them in a way that is practical and usable in everyday life.

In addition to his workshops for lay people, Dr. Dreaver is the leading chiropractic authority on Somatic Technique, an advanced method of releasing chronically tight muscles and enhancing mind/body awareness. He teaches this work to other health professionals throughout the U.S. He resides with his son in Sebastopol, California, where he maintains a private practice in both chiropractic and individual transformational work.

To Write the Author

If you wish to contact the author or would like more information about this book, please write to the author in care of Llewellyn Worldwide, and we will forward your request. Both the author and publisher appreciate hearing from you and learning of your enjoyment of this book and how it has helped you. Llewellyn Worldwide cannot guarantee that every letter written to the author can be answered, but all will be forwarded. Please write to:

Dr. Jim Dreaver
c/o Llewellyn Worldwide
P.O. Box 64383-K244, St. Paul, MN 55164-0383, U.S.A.

Please enclose a self-addressed, stamped envelope for reply or $1.00 to cover costs.
If outside the U.S.A., enclose international postal reply coupon.

Llewellyn's Whole Life Series

The
Ultimate
Cure

The Healing Energy Within You

Dr. Jim Dreaver

1996
Llewellyn Publications
P.O. Box 64383
St. Paul, Minnesota 55164-0383

Cover design by Tom Grewe
Interior editing, layout and design by Laura Gudbaur

FIRST EDITION
First Printing, 1996

The 19 lines from the *Tao Te Ching* reprinted by permission of Harper-Collins Publishers, Inc. Translation copyright © 1988 by Stephen Mitchell. The selection on pp 208-209 from *Dialogue on the Path of Initiation*, by Alphonse Goettman (Globe Press Books, 1991 copyright by Ted Nottingham, Indianapolis) is reprinted with permission of Joel Friedlander, Publisher.

Library of Congress Cataloging-In-Publication Data
Dreaver, Jim.
      The ultimate cure: the healing energy within you / Jim Dreaver
          p. cm. -- (Llewellyn's whole life series)
      Includes index.
      ISBN 1-56718-224-5 (trade pbk.)
      1. Spiritual life. 2. Spiritual healing. 3. Self-actualization (Psychology) I. Title. II. Series
      BL624.D74 1995   95-45883
      291.4'4--dc20   CIP

Llewellyn Publications
A Division of Llewellyn Worldwide, Ltd.
P.O. Box 64383-0383
St. Paul, Minnesota 55164-0383

About Llewellyn's Whole Life Series

Each of us is born into a body, but an amazing number of us lack anything beyond the most utilitarian connection with our physical beings. Yet, being "in touch" with the body—being aware of the senses' connection to our thoughts, emotions, dreams, and spirits—is integral to holistic living.

Instead of taking the intellect or the spirit as a starting point, books in the Whole Life Series focus on the physical—sensation and bodily health—and how it is inextricably linked with the health of our minds and souls.

What does the physical have to do with the emotional or the spiritual? Everything. We are as much beings of the Earth as we are beings of the stars ... our senses and connection to our bodies are just as integral to our physical, emotional, and spiritual well-being as is our connection to our higher selves.

The old doctrines, which regard the physical as inferior to the spiritual, may have made sense for the medieval ascetic—but, much like the medieval belief that the Sun orbited the Earth, those beliefs have been supplanted by more enlightened ones. Fortunately. It is impossible to truly feel that we belong in the universe, just as much as the ground we walk on and the air we breathe, until we entirely accept our own natures as physical and spiritual creatures. This book will help you heal the split between will and understanding and further your journey to wholeness, the place where body, mind, and spirit are integrated and healed. Access your internal source of wisdom, love, and healing through the techniques presented here for heightened mind and body awareness ... and become so much more than the sum of your parts.

Dedication

To Barbara, woman of spirit, who
awakened me to the beauty, mystery, and
power of the feminine, without which
there is no healing.

And to Adam, our son, who is such a
bright and wonderful light in my life.

Table of Contents

Acknowledgments

I've had the love, support, and guidance of many good people. In addition to Barbara Banes, and our son, Adam, I want to pay special tribute to my mother, Ella, and my father, Jim, for being such great parents. Thanks for being there.

My brothers, Alan and Kerry, though we live oceans apart, have always had a place in my heart.

Erich Schiffmann came into my life when I was first opening to the energy. He has long been my friend and ally. The countless hours we spent *dharma*-jousting contributed many ideas to this book.

John and Letitia Allan's friendship and love of spirit is one of the real blessings in my life. John's writings on spirituality continue to be a source of nourishment for me.

Frank and Linda Cassirer's friendship has also meant much to me. Frank's clear, luminous presence is a constant reminder of what this journey is really about.

Richard and Sheldon Murphy's generosity and love for God have made them the best of friends. They have become spiritual family.

Everyone needs a friend to whom they can say anything. Larry Elsener is that friend in my life. More than anyone else, he taught me what was needed to walk in the world with balance.

Darrell Price's clarity and quiet strength have been an important influence, as has Greg Wilson's friendship and insight into the nature of reality. I count Briar Rayne as one of the special people in my life. I value Don and Polli Schmitt, and have learned much from Don's pragmatism. Peter and Cindy Madill were there for Adam and me, and I appreciate what I've shared with Peter. The practical wisdom of Phil and Ellen Salyer has always been welcome, and I've enjoyed my connection with Phil. John Amodeo is a caring friend who has taught me much about the writer's art. Richard Miller has been a wise and steadfast companion on the spiritual journey.

I also want to acknowledge Ariel Kouros for the gifts she brought into my life; Rico Provasoli, for the professional and spiritual camaraderie we've shared through many years; Liz Callen for her commitment to awakening; Peter Davis for his impeccability; Christine DeVai for her grace; Joe and Patricia Baxter, for providing spiritual community; Web Cotton, for his compassion; and Shirley Dodds, for the light she shines in Taupo, New Zealand.

Also, Steve and Britt Gershon for their friendship, and for Steve's wry wit and wisdom; Dan Gustafson and Leslie Claire, for the stimulating dialogues we've had during the course of a long friendship; Lia Olson, for her heart; Meg Watts, for her passion; Bettie Dakotah for her energy; Matthew and Joan Greenblatt for their encouragement; Barbara Bagley for her untiring support during the years we worked together; and all my patients, and the participants in my workshops, for giving me such an extraordinary opportunity to grow in compassion and understanding.

Joyce Barnes has been a good friend and gave invaluable editorial help with the manuscript. I am especially thankful to the staff at Llewellyn for believing in this book: Nancy Mostad for seeing its merit, Lynne Menturweck for her design contribution, Tom Grewe for the striking cover, and Laura Gudbaur for her fine editing.

Most important of all, I want to acknowledge my teachers, without whom there would be no transformation to write about. I am fortunate in that I had some of the very best. Dada showed me the beauty of silence and stillness; Richard Moss awakened my sensitivity to subtle energies; Stephano Sabetti taught me to trust my power. Above all, I am indebted to the late J. Krishnamurti, whose revolutionary teachings pointed me towards the ultimate—and to Jean Klein, whose penetrating wisdom took me there.

I thank you all from the depths of my heart.

This is something most marvelous if you can come upon it.

—J. Krishnamurti

Introduction

For many years now, I've been leading workshops on healing and spirituality. Whenever I teach, I am myself healed and renewed by the experience. There's frequently an extraordinary presence in the room, a palpable energy of love and Grace. People actually feel it. At some level, they recognize the energy as pure spirit, the divine intelligence, or power, behind creation. In its own magical way, this energy touches us individually in the ways we need most. It brings us together, uniting us in our hearts, minds, and souls.

The workshops have grown out of my own healing journey, which began in 1975 with a health crisis, when I thought I was having a heart attack. I was twenty-nine. The incident put me in such a state of anxiety that for months I was afraid to go to sleep at night for fear I would lose control over my breathing and die. Eventually I realized that it was not an organic heart problem but stress. I needed to learn to slow down and get out of my head, where I had lived for too many years. I needed to come down into my feelings, my emotions, my body.

I began studying yoga, meditation, and Zen—the elusive art of living in the present. I did a lot of reading, especially the works of Krishnamurti, Herman Hesse, Alan Watts, Eugen Herrigel, and Aldous Huxley. Later I went to personal growth workshops and spiritual retreats. I explored psychotherapy as a transformational tool. I also had several spiritual teachers who came from the Eastern tradition, where the emphasis isn't on beliefs and dogma about spirituality, but on the direct experience of it.

Then, two years after that crisis, in the summer of 1977, I woke up early one morning and everything in my mind—thoughts, images, the residue of the night's dreams—dropped away. Suddenly I found myself in the most extraordinary state of clarity and stillness I had ever known. It was as if a veil had been lifted from my consciousness and I was seeing Reality for the very first time. What I saw was that everything was perfect as it was and that I was loved by God, by creation. There was no sense of separateness from anything, just a profound awareness of the fundamental unity, beauty, and sacredness of life.

Although I didn't have words for it at the time I realized that, in some way, I'd touched the source of all healing. I'd been blessed with a taste of enlightenment, of what the Zen writer, D. T. Suzuki, called "The lightning-and-thunder discovery that the universe and oneself are not remote and apart, but an intimate, palpitating Whole."

As a result of that experience, many changes have taken place in my life. My relationship with that Reality, the beauty and simplicity that is at the heart of life, has deepened and expanded. Before, I didn't know myself as a spiritual being. I had a lot of self-doubt, and often felt confused about what I was here to do. Now I feel connected to something universal, something inexhaustible that is a continuing source of nourishment and inspiration to me, no matter what problem or difficulty I may be facing.

My purpose in writing this book is to help you come to this discovery within yourself—or, if you are already in touch with it, to offer guidance in deepening the experience, so that your spirituality can become more integrated in your daily life.

Very often we get scared off by the prospect of inner work, of looking too deeply into ourselves. We may be afraid of the demons we'll discover, or the changes we may have to make in our lives. Yet we can't create change if we're afraid of change. And the demons themselves are actually illusions, perpetuated by myth and belief, by our refusal to look. The truth is that the experience of awakening is within reach of all of us. It begins to happen naturally as we learn to let go of our ego attachments, our concepts about "how" to live, and make the choice to be more present in our lives, more attuned to the subtle energy—the loving presence—that is behind creation.

It helps, too, if you can accept the view that the experience of spiritual well-being is indeed your natural state, and that there is in fact nothing spiritually to "attain." Everything you seek is already inside you. Much of the information in this book is to help you re-orient your thinking so that you can begin to trust, to accept the truth of this proposition. Once you stop striving for some ideal of spiritual perfection, there's an immense unburdening that begins to happen. The ego, in giving up its struggle for control, for some idealized state of lasting peace and security, finally grows quiet. Space opens up in the mind, and light—the illumination that has so long been sought—begins to pour in.

Listen, for example, to these words from Ramana Maharshi, a spiritual master who lived in India: "Happiness is inborn in the true Self. Your search for happiness is an unconscious search for your true Self." Jean Klein, who is from Europe, puts it this way: "True joy is not linked to outside circumstances, it flows directly from within you, from the Self." In the Christian tradition we find the same idea expressed in Jesus' teaching: "The kingdom of God is within you." Or, in the words of St. Francis of Assisi: "What you are looking for is what is looking."

These are powerful words, empowering words. When you read deeply into them, you begin to understand for yourself why the experience of spiritual awakening has been spoken of as the "ultimate cure" for human suffering. Yet what does it actually mean to be awakened? How does it look and feel in everyday life?

For me, Suzuki's definition says it as eloquently as any. Once you've had this glimpse of Reality, that you and the universe are indeed One, it starts to free you in all kinds of ways. You begin to realize that you're more than your body, mind, and emotions, more than your personality, more than the role you play in life. You begin to intuit that you're bigger than any fear, problem, or conflict you may experience. You live more and more with the awareness that there's something authentic and beautiful within you, something timeless that is the ground both of your own Being and of creation itself. And that awareness guides you in your life. You live with greater clarity, certainty, purpose. You realize, finally, why you are here, and what your work is.

Regardless of how your awakening manifests in the world, the feeling that accompanies it is always the same: it's one of increasing freedom and joy, a happiness that stands on its own. It truly is a "peace that passes all understanding." In yoga it's called *satchitananda*, a Sanskrit term which means, "the bliss that comes from the knowledge of one's true Being."

If you look back at your life, you may recall times when you've had this feeling, this sense of infinite well-being—or at least had flashes of it. They're like little enlightenments. They usually come when things quiet down a bit, when you find yourself more present, more aware, more sensitive in the moment. Anything done meditatively or contemplatively—that is, with heightened awareness—helps you get to this place where you're naturally still inside. Thoughts and images drop away and something deeper, the truth of your inner Being, begins to emerge.

This is what frequently happens in the workshops I give. My goal is to create an environment where people can get a feeling for the spiritual energy that is our true nature. Once the workshop begins my commitment is to be as present as I can be, attuned to the energy that's in the room. I invite the participants into that presence and then we allow the energy to work in its own mysterious way. The things we may do—movement, meditation, various awareness exercises, or simply engaging in open, heartfelt dialogue—are guided by the energy itself, the wisdom of the moment. It's all very natural and right. There's space enough in the room for anything to happen, and everything that happens always seems to be just what is needed.

The workshops are a constant reminder to me of what a beautiful gift it is to take a day or two out of our lives for this kind of exploration of who and what we are. It's always a rich and rewarding experience. It's a coming back Home to ourselves, to our true Selves. And what we discover, most of us, is that my Self and your Self are not so different. At the heart of things, where it matters, we really are One.

In this book I'd like to share some of the things you might learn were you to actually attend a workshop of mine. Each of the twenty-one chapters that follows represents a tool, an approach you can work with that will support you on the journey back to your Self.

Take the tools, play with them, experiment with them, find out the ways in which they might work for you. Let yourself feel the energy behind my words and you may be surprised at what begins to move within you, what new insights and feelings are awakened.

Many people who attend a workshop leave feeling a sense of centeredness, of clarity and inner peace, they haven't felt in a long time. They feel more on purpose, more directed. They come away with a greater trust in their own knowing. They feel ready to take the next step, to meet the next challenge in their lives.

Some, finding all their resistance melting, the chronic tension and anxiety within them dissolving, experience physical and emotional healing. Perhaps for the first time they feel themselves really deeply, or they see something in an entirely different way, so that it opens up a new range of possibilities for them.

Others get more in touch with their pain, their conflict. The energy of unconditional love and acceptance in the room helps bring the issues that need to be worked with more to consciousness, where they can be seen and addressed. Those looking for guidance often find out what they need to do next, how best to create the breakthrough that will free them from whatever may be holding them back.

No matter what their personal need or agenda, all come away, to some degree or other, with a sense that they're fundamentally okay as they are. They realize that the healing they seek is not so much about acquiring anything new, as it is learning to discover the depth and fullness that's already within them.

And this is my message to you. You are a beautiful human being. There may be things you need to change, or want to change, outwardly in your life—whether to do with your health, your relationships, your work, your finances, or something else—but inside, in your essence, you are *enough*, just as you are. It's important to realize this, and to remind yourself of it often. The more you trust it, the more it'll become a reality for you. It's a matter of learning to be quiet and still, and beginning to look within yourself—rather than outside—for the love and fulfillment you seek. Do this and sooner or later you'll awaken to your own innate wholeness.

You'll feel this wholeness as a current of joy, of well-being, flowing through every cell in your body. Whenever you stop and turn to it, it'll be there—not as the product of anything you think or do, but precisely because it's the substance, the very essence, of your Being. Moreover, you'll realize that this energy is in everyone and in all things. It's the exquisite pulse—the divine spark—of creation itself.

The more you touch this energy, the more you'll find all your deeper questions about life being answered. Your inner doubts and fears will begin to fall away. What will be left will be an increasing sense of ease and well-being in body, mind, and spirit. Times of tension and disturbance will continue to arise in your experience, especially during those moments when you are caught in the ego's grip, in the mental and emotional contraction that is the hallmark of self-will. But even the periods of contraction will be as ripples on the surface of the water. Underneath, in the depths of your Being, that clarity and stillness will be more and more there.

Even if there's a problem that won't go away—a health condition that seems beyond help, or some other limiting circumstance—you won't worry about it so much. You'll understand that so long as you're alive, there'll always be problems, for such is the nature of human existence. The more connected you are to the healing energy within you, the less of a "problem" such limitations become. You'll just deal with them in the most intelligent and appropriate way you can—and you'll be surprised at how perfectly everything will tend to turn out.

You'll understand that you are not your body, and that who you really are doesn't die. Instead of being afraid of death, you'll develop a deep and growing trust in the natural unfolding of life. Dying will be seen as yet another step in this endless journey your soul is on. You'll learn to welcome uncertainty, to delight in the mystery, the wonder of existence. Just as it was when you were a child, each day will again begin to feel like a new adventure to you.

With this trust will come self-acceptance, and out of self-acceptance will flow a natural acceptance of others. You'll stop wasting your energy in comparing yourself to others. You'll see the futility of judging them, of trying to "fix" or change them. You'll be happy instead with being yourself, with living your own truth. You'll realize that to express yourself in this way is the most valuable gift you can ever give anyone. Truly, it's the beginning of love—and only when there is love can real healing come about.

To find out all these things for yourself is the goal of the healing journey. It's an immensely rewarding journey, and one you can only make on your own. The answers to your problems and conflicts lie within you. Others can point the way back to the light within you—can inspire you, share with you, support you through difficult times—but no one else can do your inner work for you. You awaken the healing energy within you through your determination to find it. It is, in the end, a choice you make.

If you choose the path of consciousness and keep listening to your heart, keep bringing your attention back to the present, you'll come upon that energy, I promise. You'll discover that it's like a flame burning within you, a bright, steady flame that has always been there. At times you'll feel it as a clear, empty joy, and at others as a rich and full sense of *being*. It's the eternal "hum" of the universe, vibrating ceaselessly within and around you. The more you open to it, the more you'll feel it—healing you, renewing you, guiding you, sustaining you.

This energy, you'll discover, is the source of everything you've been looking for in your life. It really is the ultimate cure for whatever may be ailing you. It's the energy of your aliveness. It's the wellspring of your creativity. It's your passion, it's your joy. It's your ability to think, to dream, to laugh, to feel, and to cry. It's your spiritual essence. It's the love you've longed for all your life. It's who and what you most fundamentally are.

The energy of spirit is real. It is always here. Be still, open your mind and heart, feel it. Allow its peace and beauty to shine through you in your meetings with others. This is the way to always have it yourself.

Jim Dreaver, D.C.
Sebastopol, California

Always remember that the happiness you seek is within you. No matter what path you take, no matter how far you journey, life is going to remind you of this again and again, until the day comes when you finally understand and begin to relax into the peace and fullness of your own Being.

Chapter 1
Look Within

Many years ago, during one of the first workshops I ever gave, I asked one of the women present what she was looking for in her life and she responded by saying, "Inner peace."

Her reply struck me. I knew she meant it and I knew that, at some level, it was the healing all of us in that workshop were seeking. Certainly, the search for inner peace, for a deep spiritual well-being, had been a driving force in my own life ever since I was young and had sought release from the tensions and conflicts I experienced as a child.

What is necessary for this inner peace, this spiritual healing, to come about? How do you find it? Is it even attainable, given the responsibilities most of us have, the fast-paced, competitive world we live in? The great spiritual traditions, both of the East and West, assure us that it's possible to have inner peace, even while involved in daily life, in raising a family, working at a job, and so on. They speak of certain conditions for finding it, such as non-attachment to the things of the material world; surrender of the ego to a deeper knowing, to God; and love, or compassion, for self and others.

My own path has tended to be non-traditional. I've always had a problem with formal religions, starting with the one I was raised in. God was something very personal to me, and didn't seem to have a lot to do with going to church on Sunday and practicing what were for me empty rituals. Nor could I ever buy into the argument that there was only one "true" religion or way—or that you needed an agent, a priest, a "savior," to experience God. Perhaps it was inevitable that the spiritual teachers who came into my life and helped guide my way were also non-traditional.

There's an old saying, however: "At the end of all paths, there I wait." As I've continued to follow my inner guidance, I've developed an increasing appreciation for the beauty and truth of my Western spiritual heritage. Perhaps many of us needed to leave the tradition we were raised in in order to find something real in our lives, something that traditional religion was originally intended to help us find. It's like the teenager who rebels, perhaps even flees the home, in order to find him or herself. Only later, when real maturity has begun to be attained, can he or she rediscover the love that has always been there, deep inside, for the parents.

When I first contemplated the traditional spiritual ideals of non-attachment, surrender, and compassion, they seemed quite unattainable to me. There were times when I could feel compassion for others, but I was definitely very attached to things, especially to my beliefs and opinions, and I was also willful and headstrong. The word "surrender" was anathema to me. It spoke of passivity, weakness, powerlessness—the exact opposite of all the qualities that I wanted to manifest!

Nevertheless, the quest for inner peace continued to push me on. Life, the great teacher, gradually began to show me the inevitable limits of my ego, of asserting my personal will. I learned that the more I tried to push the river, go against the natural flow of events, the more frustration and unhappiness I suffered. Then there were personal losses. There were some big ones, such as divorce and financial misfortune, and many little ones along the way, and they taught me something about non-attachment. Even my beliefs about life, I noticed, dropped away or were replaced as my experience changed. Just like the Buddhists said, nothing—no "thing"—lasted forever. They even had a word for it—*anicca*, impermanence. It's one of the key tenets of Buddhist philosophy.

Yet through all these changes, "I" was still here. "I"—this awareness, or consciousness that I am—continued to survive it all. "Discover who that 'I' is," one of my teachers said to me, "and you will find the peace you are looking for."

This is surely the great spiritual teaching of all time, the one affirmed by Socrates: "Know thyself." Yet what is the path to self-knowing? In many ways, this whole book is about the journey of self-knowing. Through learning to be in your body, to develop your sensitivity, to meditate, to heal your relationships, to find out what you love to do—through all these approaches and ways of being you get to know yourself as a multi-dimensional, spiritually-alive human being.

The Limits of Intellectual Understanding

True self-knowing has nothing to do with intellectual constructs, nor does it depend upon ideals, beliefs, or theories. Indeed, such concepts only get in the way of authentic spiritual experience, although it takes most of us years to appreciate this—especially if we have a tendency to over-intellectualize, to live in our heads!

Speaking for myself, I spent a long time trying to "understand" life intellectually, trying to get a mental grip on it. I was convinced that once I had the conceptual "answer," or solution, to a problem—especially concerning the nature of happiness and suffering—then I'd be free to live my life without conflict. With the right attitude, I believed, it would be a fairly simple matter to minimize my suffering and maximize my happiness at all times in the future.

Not so! No matter how often I thought I'd "found" the answer, I could never seem to hold onto happiness, and nor could I avoid suffering. In fact, the more I clung to my "answers," my theories, the more I seemed to suffer! Eventually I discovered that every new conflict, every new problem, required its own fresh response. Life was carrying me to new and deeper levels within myself, places within my heart and my psyche where the old answers didn't apply anymore. This is why, today, I can appreciate the words of the Sufi teacher, Idries Shah, when he says, "No matter what point of truth or understanding you arrive at, there is always one beyond it." This piece of wisdom, more than any other, helped me get free of my attachment to conceptual understanding.

There came a time in my own healing journey when I began to work with teachers, like Jean Klein, who had gone beyond concepts, who knew that truth didn't lie in words or beliefs. They appreciated that living was essentially a non-linear, non-rational experience. There was a place for linear thinking, for reason, logic, and analysis. This type of thinking, which is often termed left-brained, or masculine thinking, was especially useful when dealing with objective physical reality, with "things"—such as economics, technology, and logistical planning—that were at least somewhat subject to human control.

But when you are dealing with matters of the heart, with the healing of emotional suffering and the quest for meaning and fulfillment in life, a different approach is needed. Control doesn't work here. In fact, it often runs counter to the innate wisdom of life. In the realm of the heart, it is the feminine, or right-brained, qualities of feeling, trust, and intuition that are important. Understanding this dance between the masculine and feminine is so essential to emotional well-being that I've given it a chapter of its own later in this book.

Learning to Work Directly with Energy

The teachers I studied with were masters, in that they were able to work directly with these subtler energies. What they taught didn't rely upon a conceptual framework. They knew there was no "model," no blueprint for being a whole and integrated person. Their own masculine and feminine energies were well-balanced. They knew how to accomplish things in the world. Above all, they knew how to *be*. They were fundamentally at ease and content within themselves, no matter what was going on externally, and they had a delightful spontaneity about them, a creativity that was often surprising in its originality. In this sense they were true artists, artists in the most difficult art of all— the art of living happily and successfully.

Needless to say, I wanted what they had. I, myself, was pretty well burned-out on sophisticated psychological theories and clever metaphysical concepts. I'd been doing battle with my mind for a long time and it seemed I'd exhausted the possibilities for finding any lasting happiness through intellectual understanding. What I was looking for now was not an idea or belief, but an *experience*. I wanted the experience of feeling joyful and peaceful inside. I wanted the experience of being confident and focused in my actions. I wanted the experience of feeling loved.

Irina Tweedie, an elderly and delightful English spiritual teacher, gives a wonderful account of her work with a Sufi master in her book, *Chasm Of Fire*. In the book she quotes her master, who says, "We do not teach, we quicken. I am stronger than you so your currents adjust themselves to mine. This is a simple law of nature. The stronger current will affect, quicken, the weaker."

This was precisely what happened when I was in the presence of my teachers. They were much clearer, more present, more in touch with something essential in life than I was. When I was around them, my own consciousness expanded. I felt more whole, more my true Self. I had the experience of being quickened, healed at many levels of my being. I could literally feel a new energy stirring inside me.

Whatever your spiritual path, you'll find, if it's a true path, that it will bring you to this place. You'll be freer of concepts and beliefs, and you'll live more and more out of an energy, a feeling, within you. A feeling of clarity, of harmony, of a growing sense of confidence and creative power, the power that you feel when you're connected to something infinitely bigger than yourself.

It's this feeling of inner well-being—even though you may only touch it in moments at first—that gives rise to the "knowing" of your real Self. The knowing is something intuited. You begin to realize that there's a divine wisdom behind everything, an energy of love and goodness that is guiding you on your journey through life. You know it because you *feel* it, just as you know you're hungry because you feel it. And out of this knowing arises a profound sense of trust.

At the same time you'll find that what you know can't readily be put into words. To describe the nature of enlightenment, of that inner joy that depends on nothing outside itself, is very difficult to do. The spiritual, or unitive experience, with its feeling of immensity and timelessness, of pure emptiness and all-pervading fullness, doesn't translate easily into the language of the ordinary, everyday world. Yet when you're in touch with the source energy, the ground of Being, when you can smell the fragrance of it, the right words will come to you should you ever need them.

What brings you to the source is the path you take. Don Juan, Carlos Castaneda's spiritual teacher, said that it didn't matter what path you chose, so long as it had a heart. There's great truth in this, for the path with a heart always leads you back to what's inside your own heart. You end up with more and more of yourself—your true Self.

Meditation

Whatever path you take (and you'll undoubtedly travel down many roads during your life's journey), you'll find that it will likely involve some form of meditation, for it's meditation that teaches you to look within. It's through meditation that you get beyond your mind and its conceptual limitations into the realm of genuine spiritual experience. I doubt there is anyone who has ever awakened to their spiritual nature—and, even more important, been able to embody that experience so that it becomes a living reality for them—without spending time in meditation, or contemplation.

There's a chapter in this book devoted entirely to meditation and how to go about it, but because it's so basic to the healing journey, I want to introduce the subject here. In its simplest definition, meditation is communion with spirit, or the divine. It's learning to sit and tune in to yourself—and what is around you—so that you can begin to awaken to the underlying unity and beauty of life.

On the way to the discovery of that unity, you'll almost certainly encounter a good deal of emotional pain and fear. This is the dark, or "shadow," side of your psyche which, until you make the commitment to self-knowing, you'll usually do everything you can to avoid. This is normal. None of us likes being uncomfortable. It's easy to enjoy meditating when it feels blissful or peaceful, but when we start to get restless, bored, or agitated in some way, it's another story!

Meditation, provided you don't get caught in some mechanical technique or practice, will make you more sensitive to life, to feeling. When you sit in stillness and silence, which is the essence of meditation, your awareness begins to expand naturally. You start to notice more, to see more, to hear more, to feel more—both externally, in your environment, and internally, in your own body, mind, and soul. It's this growing sensitivity that is the double-edged sword in meditation. Too often it'll become more than you're willing to handle—yet handle it you must, if you want to be free of the conflicting thoughts and images, the mental chatter, that distracts you from the experience of your true Self.

The Balance between Control and Surrender

How then do you live with increasing sensitivity? This is where will, or personal power, plays a vital role. You must learn to be really present with whatever you're experiencing. You must be as strong as possible in your body, which is why diet and exercise are so important on this journey. Paying attention to your physical health helps you stay grounded and centered.

Spiritual seekers often make the mistake of thinking that they have to dissolve their ego and so assume a kind of passivity in the way they deal with life. When things start to heat up, when the energies, the feelings, the emotions get intense—whether in meditation, in their relationships, or in some other area of life—they can't handle it. They're not present enough. They've given up their personal power in the mistaken belief that they must meekly accept whatever happens to them.

Remember, you can't "dissolve" your own ego. To even begin to think you can is a very egotistical notion! All you can do is surrender, or align yourself, with whatever is happening in the moment. This means letting go of thought, of analytical thinking, and bringing your attention into the present. The more aware you are in your body, the easier it is to then deal with whatever may come up. To surrender in this way is not the same as being passive. Passivity is collapse, despair. It's to allow yourself to be swept along helplessly—and eventually overwhelmed by—forces that seem beyond your control.

True surrender is bringing yourself fully and consciously into the here-and-now. It is moving *with* the current of life, without being drowned in it. It's learning to dance with the energy, to blend with it, to flow with it, but not to lose the sense of yourself as an individual self, or entity. In true surrender you become a spiritual warrior. You become a participant, a co-creator with life, with God. You don't become a helpless victim.

Finding that balance between control and surrender, between knowing when to hold on and when to let go, is one of the main tasks on the spiritual journey. A friend of mine described this process as "the dance of Grace and will." Too much control, and the healing energy of Grace, with all its potential to bring about something fresh and new in your life, is blocked. Too much letting go, on the other hand, can lead to indecisiveness and ineffectiveness, so that it becomes difficult to do anything productive and meaningful.

The balance, as you might guess, lies in the middle. It really is a dance. It's a matter of being able to remain fluid, open, and sensitive to the flow of events and yet all the while be awake and alert, so that you can act decisively and creatively when needed. It's to be present with your whole Being, which means not just your ego, your personal will, but also your intuition, your higher Self.

The Role of Will and Intention

You begin to see, then, where will and intentionality fit in the spiritual perspective. They are functions of your spirituality, expressions of your higher Self. Spiritual work, meditation, develops the all-important quality of impersonality within you. It's the impersonality that allows you to be detached from the fruits of your actions. This detachment frees you up to respond in the most appropriate way to the challenges confronting you. It's the impersonality that allows you to see the big picture, the widest possible perspective. It's the impersonality that allows you to feel compassion for all people, all life, and not just play favorites.

In a person who is developed spiritually, however, the impersonal always expresses itself in a very personal way. There's still an ego there, a healthy, developed sense of an individual "I" or self, but the difference is that the personal element doesn't get in the way.

As you awaken spiritually, your ego becomes more transparent. You still have an "I," a "me," but the difference now is that you realize you're not separate from all the other "I's" in the world. You draw your inspiration from something much larger than yourself—from God, the source. You live more and more from the fundamental spiritual truth: *"I am the universe, and the universe is me."* It's only when you're still asleep spiritually that you believe yourself to be separate and alone, distant from God, and unrelated to the rest of the universe. It's this feeling of separateness, of aloneness and isolation, that is behind the anxiety and insecurity your personal self feels.

Until you wake up to the truth of who you are, of your oneness with spirit, you remain unenlightened. You continue to live, like most human beings, in a kind of existential darkness, a state of hypnotism, or mesmerism. That's the way it's meant to be. You're here to discover, through your inner work, who you really are and how best to live. The suffering you endure helps you wake up, points you back to truth, to the need for meditation, self-reflection, inquiry. While it's foolish to want to suffer, when suffering does come into your life, it's wise to pay close attention to it.

Suffering can be a powerful teacher. It's the signal, the warning bell, that lets you know it's time to look anew at how you're dealing with life. As Jean Klein once remarked, fortunate is the person for whom the bell tolls loudly. It's only the prolonged suffering, the conflict that gnaws away at you but never gets quite acute enough to stir you into action, that wears you down and makes you ill and unhappy.

As you go deeper with your meditation and, especially, bring that quality of meditative awareness into every dimension of your life, you'll realize the truth of all these things for yourself. You'll discover the role of will and intention. You'll see how important it is to not give away your power—to not relinquish your own unique, God-given Selfhood to any outside force or influence, whether it be a blissful experience, a seductive belief or idea, a controlling or rigid organization, or a charismatic *guru* or teacher.

While you'll learn much from observing your environment and listening to others, you'll also learn to discriminate. You'll take in what is useful to you and you'll discard the rest. In time, you'll come to realize that the surrender required of you is not to an idea, feeling, or experience, not to a person, teaching, or institution, but to the creative principle of life itself, the boundless energy that is to be found in the depths of your own Being.

Self-Acceptance

When you start to become really present in your meditation, so that you're not using it to escape from reality or get lost in bliss, then it leads naturally to self-acceptance. Self-acceptance is the great peace-maker—so important that it, too, is given a chapter of its own in the pages that follow. It's a beautiful moment when you finally stop fighting yourself and can look at your reflection in the mirror, and for the first time feel truly at peace with what you see.

As one of my favorite fortune cookies says, "Be kind. Every man you meet is fighting a hard battle." That kindness starts within, with the acceptance of your imperfections, your shortcomings, your humanness. It's when you are gentle with yourself that you really begin to feel compassion for others. No one is perfect. Even the most spiritually-evolved individuals are still human. They get sick, they occasionally get into fights or arguments with their associates, they make mistakes, they sometimes have unhealthy habits like smoking or drinking, and they even worry at times (though never for very long) about money and paying bills.

One of the traps on the spiritual path is the tendency we often have to want to attach ourselves to a teacher or *guru* who seems to embody the qualities—such as wisdom, strength, kindness—that we feel we lack. It's one thing to admire and learn from another human being, but to put someone on a pedestal and regard him or her as infallible is proof that we don't yet know ourselves. It shows that we're not yet at ease with our own humanness. Looking to an out-side authority, especially in spiritual matters, is one of the main ways we disempower ourselves. We literally give our power away, usually out of our emotional hunger for the perfect father or mother figure that we never had when we were children.

You have to find the strength of the father and the love of the mother within you. That's a good deal of what awakening is all about. That's where self-acceptance leads. It brings you to the place where you no longer judge yourself for your shortcomings. Or, if you're still inclined to judge yourself, then you no longer judge yourself so severely for having such judgments!

Once you start to come to this place, it's tremendously empowering. You're no longer dissipating your energy in conflict and self-condemnation. You begin to feel more of a sense of wholeness and ease within. You get an appreciation for your own divinity, your own innate goodness. In this way you come to discover that you are the world and the world is you. You realize that the well-being you're beginning to feel within is nothing other than your personal experience of the innate perfection of life—the beautiful mystery of creation that the ancient Chinese philosopher, Lao Tzu, called the Tao, the Zen masters Buddha-nature, and the Christian mystics Grace, or the Holy Spirit.

When you commit yourself to spiritual awakening, it sooner or later brings you to the realization of all this. The net result of the work you do, the suffering you go through, the doubt and uncertainty, the failed efforts and unsuccessful attempts, is that you come through it all with a richer and fuller sense of your Self—and a greater appreciation for this gift, this extraordinary adventure called *Life*.

Learning to breathe slowly and consciously clears your mind, relaxes your body, and helps you experience a deeper emotional and spiritual well-being.

Chapter 2
Breathe!

The first practical step toward awakening the healing energy within you is learning to be more centered and relaxed in your body. Centering, in turn, begins with the art of conscious breathing. In my workshops and in my healing practice the most important exercise I give people is to remind them to *breathe*, to continually come back to their breath as a way of keeping their energy flowing and helping them stay grounded and present.

I discovered a long time ago, through my own yoga practice and related awareness exercises, that the more relaxed and comfortable I was in my body, the easier it was for my busy mind to slow down. The more my mind slowed down, the more space there was between my thoughts. As space opened up in my mind, new awarenesses, new perceptions began to reveal themselves to me. In this way I began to have deeper and more lasting experiences of the energy of love and wholeness which is always there, under the surface of things.

It's no accident that one of the foundational practices in just about all Eastern spiritual disciplines is conscious breathing—using the breath as a vehicle for quieting the mind and bringing one's awareness more fully into the present. The words "breath" and "spirit" have the same Latin root. The very first thing we did when we came into this world was take a deep breath. We literally "inspired" ourselves into life. The very last thing we'll do is let our breath go. Death is the final act of "expiration" as our spirit, who we really are, lets go of our body and merges once more with the universal ground of Being, our spiritual Home.

I remember a powerful dream I had some years ago in which the significance of the breath was brought home to me most graphically. In the dream I was receiving a teaching about dying. I wasn't dying, but I was aware that one day I would die, and that there was something important I needed to remember in order to be able to face my death without fear.

The teaching was coming from my higher Self and it spoke to me with these words: "Just remember, *breathe*. That's all you have to do. Take one last, deep, conscious breath, let it go gently, and everything will be okay." It was a beautiful dream and it took away a lot of the fears I'd had about dying. Now I knew how to let go, to make my transition—when the time came—in the most effortless, painless way possible. All I had to do was remember to breathe, and simply relax, let go, into the waiting presence of God.

Breath as the Key to Life and Health

At the same time, I realized, I was being given a teaching about life, about how to live. Breathing was the key there, too. It was the way to deal with all fears. The more deeply you breathe, the more life you take in. To inhale fully is to say "Yes" to life with your whole being. It's to empower yourself through embracing the totality of the moment. It's to reconnect with your spiritual Self, to affirm your oneness with universal wisdom, the source of your creativity and your intelligence.

To exhale completely, on the other hand, is to let go of everything you hold onto inwardly—all tension, thoughts, worries.

Through exhalation the old is emptied out, creating space, making way for the new. Exhalation is an act of surrender, of trust, of faith. It's an act of courage.

To breathe in anew is to be reborn. To fully let go of the breath is, in a very real sense, a dying to the moment. In learning to breathe consciously in this way you find yourself gradually getting freer of the fear of dying itself. You begin to understand the secret of life—that it's a continuum, and that while your body will some day fall away, like a suit of clothes you have outgrown, life itself, your essential nature, is eternal.

Your breath is the connecting link between your conscious mind and the many unconscious processes that keep your body functioning at an optimal level. Breathing itself is an act which happens unconsciously, automatically, yet it's also one you can readily bring under conscious control. Through learning to work with your own breathing, making a conscious process out of it, you can affect many of the unconscious functions in your body in a positive way.

Slowing down the breathing, for instance, slows the heart rate. It brings about a general relaxation of all internal body functions, including a lowering of blood pressure. When you're anxious, nervous, or stressed, you'll tend to breathe in a very constricted way. Your breathing will be rapid and shallow. It won't go deeper than the upper part of your chest.

People who live in a chronic state of tension, and who breathe like this as a matter of habit, fall prey to a variety of health problems. Good breathing is vital to the elimination of toxins from the body, and for proper oxygenation of the blood. It also allows for maximum diaphragmatic movement. The expansion of the diaphragm massages and moves energy through all the internal organs of the body, keeping them in a state of well-being. Chronically shallow breathing, on the other hand, limits diaphragmatic movement. It leads to respiratory problems, heart palpitations, digestive upsets, poor elimination and circulation, as well as fatigue, nervousness, and low energy states. People who think too much tend to breath too shallowly. Their energy gets "stuck" in the upper part of their body, and this makes them unbalanced, ungrounded.

Notice the tendency you may have to hold onto your breath, to restrict your breathing and thus limit the amount of energy you allow in. Learn to breathe deeply and consciously as a way of clearing your energy. It's almost impossible to be in a contracted state, to feel anxiety, fear, resentment, or any other negative emotion so long as you're breathing slowly, consciously, deeply.

The Art of Conscious Breathing

A full breath begins with exhalation, with gently pulling in your belly as you breathe out. This forces your diaphragm upwards, naturally expelling the air from your lungs. If you do this properly, you don't have to work at inhaling. It happens spontaneously. Your belly relaxes and expands. It pulls down on your diaphragm, causing an inrush of fresh oxygen. Then you should let your rib cage and chest open up, and your shoulders rise so that your lungs can fill with air. Pause briefly, then allow the process to begin all over again with conscious exhalation.

In Zen and other spiritual traditions, watching or following the breath is emphasized because it both focuses your attention and helps you get more centered and relaxed in your body. You can't have your attention in two places at once. When you're watching your breath, you can't at the same time be caught up in your thoughts. To focus on your breathing, then, is one of the simplest and most effective techniques for getting free of the distracting chatter of the mind.

Working with your breath as a way of getting out of your mind and into a deeper state of awareness, is made easier if you consciously slow your breathing down. Normally you breathe, or inhale, around 14–16 times per minute. You can safely reduce this frequency to 8 or 10 breaths per minute by making a meditative practice of it. Sit down in a comfortable, congenial place, either on a cushion on the floor, or on a chair. Let your back be straight, your jaw, neck, and shoulders relaxed, your hands resting loosely on your thighs or in your lap.

Now, close your eyes and begin to follow the flow of your breath. Lengthen the inhalation so that it's longer than usual. Then pause, feeling into the stillness at the end of the breath. Then gently and slowly exhale. Try and make the exhalation a little longer than the inhalation. At the end of the exhalation, pause again. Once more, allow yourself to feel into the stillness, the deeper energy that begins to unfold. Don't look for any particular state or feeling. Just notice the quality of sensation, of awareness, that is present. And then begin to inhale again. You'll find this a very easy practice. If you've never meditated before, this is the perfect way to get into it.

Learn to slow your breath down in the way that I've shown you here, and you'll notice immediate benefits in terms of a more relaxed body, a clearer mind, and a more confident, trusting sense of yourself. As your awareness of your breath deepens you'll become more sensitive to the pauses, the silences in between each cycle of inhalation and exhalation. You'll begin to perceive, in those silences, that quality of wholeness, of peace and harmony, of which I've spoken.

You'll begin to actually feel, and discern for yourself, the spiritual energy that underlies and gives rise to your breath—and, indeed, your very existence.

Your body is a mirror for your relationship with the world. The more at ease you are in your body, the more at ease you'll be in your relationships, your work, in every aspect of your life.

Chapter 3
Love Your Body

Conscious breathing helps bring you into your body, into your here-and-now experience. The next step is to begin to really feel yourself in your body, to feel your aliveness, your energy, your physicality. It's to be very attuned to your body, to start to treat it as your friend, your closest ally. It's to learn to check in with your body frequently—to feel it, sense it, notice it—so that you can find out how it's doing, what it has to tell you, and what it may need.

Your body is the vehicle for your spirit and, just like your automobile, the more smoothly and efficiently it functions, the more able you are to enjoy the ride. If, on the other hand, your vehicle is always breaking down and giving trouble, it's difficult to relax and enjoy the journey. You'll always be worrying about what calamity may befall you next.

As a health practitioner, I frequently see people who literally don't live in their bodies, or at least are seldom very present in them.

They don't feel the contraction and relaxation of their muscles, the glide of their joints, the rhythm of their movement when they walk, sit, stand, or change their posture in any given way. They aren't attuned to what the late Thomas Hanna, a pioneer in the field of body/mind education and another of my mentors, termed their *somatic* experience. They don't have a keen and vibrant awareness of themselves as a living, breathing, moving, self-sensing organism.

In this high-tech, information-oriented age, it's all too easy to get caught up in your mind, your head, preoccupied with your worries, your concerns, your daydreams, your wishful-thinking. Very often, if you stop to notice it, you may realize that your attention has been somewhere else altogether, not really here at all. Your body can all too readily become just another object, like your car, your stereo, your refrigerator—something worthy of occasional notice, perhaps, but still basically an object, separate and apart from the real "you."

And yet the real "you" is your body. As the German philosopher Karlfried Graf Durckheim says in his book, *The Call For The Master*, "A person is real in the here-and-now only in a bodily form. Our bodily form is 'right' when it allows Being to *show through* as true nature—when the body is seen not as something people have but as something they are, as the sum total of gestures in which they live themselves out, in which they express and realize themselves in a visible, external form."

This is why the most valuable spiritual and psychotherapeutic disciplines have as their focus a body-based awareness of experience. Approaches like psychoanalysis—or any number of philosophical "systems" like existentialism, for example—deal in the realm of concepts and beliefs, with the intellectual understanding of experience. In doing this they reinforce the idea of an ego, a subjective "self" that exists apart from—and superior to—the body it inhabits. When people take the intellectual, or rational path, alone as a way of solving the problems in their life, they're unlikely to experience any genuine sense of personal liberation. On the contrary, they tend to remain caught in a conceptual—and increasingly "self"-centered—trap.

A genuinely transformational approach to healing the psyche brings people into their bodies. It may not involve any formalized pattern of exercise or movement, but it emphasizes the need for a sensitive awareness of the body—and to the immediate physical environment which, metaphorically, is but a larger extension of the individual physical organism. Watch a Zen master walking through a garden, and you'll see someone at ease in his or her body, someone who moves with grace and alertness, whose every step demonstrates an alive sense of relationship with the path, the air, the rocks, the plants, with every feature of the surrounding environment.

Your Body Reflects What is Happening in Your Life

When you don't have this kind of relationship with your body and the space you occupy, you're always at risk for accidents. Accidents of just about any kind—stumbling or tripping, bumping into and dropping things, making frequent mistakes—are usually the result of inattention, of unconsciousness. The next time you have an accident, try and recall what you were thinking about immediately before the incident occurred. Chances are you'll discover you were "off" in your head somewhere, caught up in a distracting thought, a memory, a daydream. Or perhaps you were feeling contracted, angry, or just worried about something. Almost certainly, you weren't present to the moment at hand.

Your body also tends to get sick much more easily when you're not present in it. You can think of your body as being like a garden. If you don't give your garden a lot of attention, watering it and feeding it regularly, nurturing it with love and care, it'll begin to die. This same process is true of your body, especially as you get older. When you're young, in your teens and twenties, you can neglect your health without, often, any serious consequences. The life force is so strong and vital it readily repels any pollutants or other obstacles to well-being. But as you move into your thirties and beyond the price of neglect becomes increasingly apparent, and sometimes the damage caused by lack of care and attention can be irreparable.

In my healing practice I see over and over again that the people with the most health problems are the ones who are least "in" their bodies. They treat their body as an object, as a nuisance almost, and have only the most superficial relationship with it.

Interestingly, Durckheim defines a neurotic as a "person who cannot find himself in his body."

It's a commonly held perspective in holistic health circles that the body gets sick in order to get our attention. My personal experience bears this out. The evidence shows over and over again that the healthiest people are those who listen to—and heed—the warning signs their body is giving them. When they feel their body is getting out of balance, or in need of some special attention, they respond with love and care, just as they would to a friend in need. They have a dynamic, loving relationship with their body.

You may notice that the more you struggle with being centered and at ease in your body, the more you probably find yourself struggling in your dealings with the world, with handling everyday things like relationships, work, money, and other responsibilities. People with unhealed emotional wounds, who daydream or fantasize a lot, or who seek out spiritual experiences as an escape from having to deal with the mundane realities of living, feel this struggle most acutely.

Facing this struggle and healing the split between your body and your inner self, that in you which longs for freedom, for wholeness, is essential for spiritual well-being. It's learning to appreciate, just like the Zen master, that the physical environment you interact with is not different or separate from the body you live in, and that your spirit, your life energy, is the mediating force. You have to learn to bring the two together. You have to learn to find God—that energy of joy, of passion, of creativity—in everyday existence, not just in special times of meditation or worship. The state of your body often closely reflects the state of your life. It truly is a mirror—a metaphor—for the way you're living.

There's a Tibetan text, *The Great Path Of Awakening*, by Jamgon Kongtrul (Shambala, translated by Ken McCleod), which says it most eloquently:

To see what you've done, look at your body.
To see what you'll be, look at your actions.

An Exercise for Heightening Physical Awareness

It's a challenge to stay in our bodies in these times because of the excessive amount of stimulation, of sensory input, to which we're all subjected. We're constantly being bombarded with all kinds of stimuli that grab at our awareness, and pull us away from the experience of what we're sensing and feeling in the here-and-now. Television, telephones, radios, newspapers, and computers are major sources of such stimulation. If on top of these you add noise pollution, the people in your life who are continually placing demands upon you, *and* the numerous commitments and responsibilities you've already got, you can see that there are myriad distracting influences diverting your attention outward, away from your natural, body-based awareness.

It's often impossible, if not impractical, to block out or eliminate all forms of stimulation from your life. Much of it you need in varying degrees in order to be able to function successfully in the world, and there's something in all of us that thrives on healthy, creative forms of stimulation anyway. But it's possible, with awareness, to not be so affected by it all. Learning to be really present in your body helps you attain a quality of freedom and detachment, so that you live more from your own center, your own inner clarity, rather than being constantly jerked about by the circumstances or chaos around you.

It's a matter of learning to relax, to be loose in your body, and yet to be keenly alert too, so that you're present with your whole being, with all of your senses. When your awareness is body-based in this way—that is, centered in your physicality, in what G. I. Gurdjieff, the Russian mystic, called the *moving* center—then you're naturally more confident and at ease with yourself. You're in touch with your physical power, your strength—and, out of that, your own inner wisdom.

A good exercise to help with developing this awareness is to stand with your feet shoulder width apart, arms hanging by your side. Wiggle your toes, rock back and forth on your soles and your heels, and establish a solid contact with the ground. This helps you stand your ground, which allows you to deal more effectively with any upset you may be experiencing within yourself. It helps you respond better to confrontational energies from outside, such as the negativity or anger of another person.

Then make sure your knees are unlocked. The conditioned tendency is to lock your knees, to literally "brace" yourself in order to ward off those real or imagined threats. This causes you to be stiff, rigid, easily thrown off-balance. When you unlock your knees, you're more flexible. With your feet planted and your knees unlocked you become like the bamboo that is firmly rooted in the earth, yet is able to bend and sway before even the fiercest wind.

Now breathe down into your belly, into the place that the Japanese call the *hara*, a couple of inches below the navel. This is your physical center of gravity, Gurdjieff's moving center. Martial artists learn how to stay centered in the *hara*. You too will find that as you learn to bring your awareness there, rather than being in your head, in thinking, it'll be very difficult for anyone to unbalance you, either physically or psychically.

The next part of this exercise is to shake out your arms and hands and let go of any tension in your shoulders. Then roll your head a few times in each direction to help eliminate any holding in the muscles there. Next your jaw. A lot of people hold tension in the jaw, and with it much anger and sadness. Open and close your mouth as wide as you can several times. Let your jaw hang a little bit loose.

Now bring your awareness earthward, back to the ground you stand on. Be aware of the space your body occupies. Look around you. Be as present as you can be in your environment. Notice the strength you draw from the earth, from the feeling of something solid, immovable, below you. Send your breath, your energy, all the way down into the ground, deep into the earth. Notice how centered, how "grounded" you feel. Notice what it's like to experience this feeling, how good it feels. The more grounded and centered you are, the easier it is to deal with any challenge that comes your way. Then you can respond intelligently to the crises of life, rather than react in a panic.

Practice this exercise several times a day as a way of developing a conscious, enlightened relationship with your body. If it's difficult for you to be in your body, whether because of pain or tension, or simply because you've been out of touch with it too long, then you may need some bodywork to help you get back "in." Chiropractic, massage, acupressure, Rolfing, and similar body therapies are all good tools for helping you become more attuned to your body so that you experience a heightened sense of physical well-being.

Dealing with Illness

Some final words on what it means to love your body: if you're presently suffering from an illness or other physical limitation, being in your body may not be very easy for you. You may just be too uncomfortable physically. If this is the case, do the best you can. If nothing else, the practice of deep, slow breathing, along with a conscious effort to feel yourself more fully in every aspect of your body, will often be effective in alleviating, or at least reducing, stress and pain.

It helps also to not fight the pain, but rather to soften around it, to give it space. When you give space like this—through accepting rather than resisting what you're experiencing, through visualizing space, expansiveness, around the problem area—there's room for the contracted energy of the pain to unwind. Given enough room, it'll often dissolve altogether.

A good technique here is to bring your awareness to the areas in your body that feel reasonably good, that feel open and light, and focus on them. Then see if you can allow the feeling of lightness to expand, so that it starts to penetrate the tighter, more painful areas. This is a practical way of learning to soften around the painful, dense places within you.

Stephen Levine, an American writer and meditation teacher, advises people to practice "softening the belly." Much tension gets held in the belly, which is the somatic center of the will, the personal self. This tension tends to radiate out and create tightness and pain throughout the rest of the body. Feeling the tension in your belly and then consciously softening it helps you let go of the contracted "me" sense, and brings about an expansion in consciousness, and a new sense of ease.

It's easier to relax your belly—or any other tight area—if you first consciously *tighten* it. Intensifying the contraction in this way brings it more into your awareness. You first have to know you *have* a problem before you can begin to let it go. Doing a practice such as this teaches you how to work with and actually control the flow of your own internal energy. The more you practice, the more quickly you'll be able to move through times of "stuckness" and contraction.

In the end, good physical health is not a prerequisite for finding inner peace and spiritual well-being. The split between body and psyche needs to be healed, yes. Your awareness needs to be brought down into your body, so that you become more sensitive to what you're feeling and experiencing in your physical reality.

But the real healing is in the heart, mind, and spirit. As you allow yourself to become more relaxed inwardly, you'll find a lot of stress and tension leaving your body. You may still have to deal with the effects of an incurable illness or disease, but you will not be so taken over or consumed by them.

Underneath whatever phenomena you may be experiencing physically, you'll become more and more aware of the energy of peace and fullness that is the real "you." You'll touch it in moments of stillness, of silence, of genuine inner quiet. As you learn to deepen your contact with this energy, your body and its pain won't be the burden it once was. You won't be so identified with it. You'll be more in harmony with the physical changes that will continue to happen throughout your life. Having learned to love and really be in your body, you'll awaken to an increasing sense of freedom from it.

In that freedom you'll become more aware of your true spiritual nature—and it's here, as you learn to trust and relax into that truth, that you'll find the deepest and most enduring well-being.

Mastering the art of conscious movement is one of the best ways of keeping the life energy flowing through you—the energy that will keep you feeling young, vibrant, healthy.

Chapter 4
Move!

To be in your body means above all to be aware of *movement*. Life is movement—and movement is life. Thomas Hanna, in his somatic work, defined reality as "things moving." Modern quantum physics teaches us that even a solid object, such as a table, is actually a collection of electrons and particles in constant motion. The healthy body is itself a dynamic, moving organism, or "thing." As Hanna pointed out, when awareness is truly awake and centered in the body, the body moves easily and effortlessly, is supple and flexible.

For years now, whenever I've felt myself getting fragmented, disconnected from my inner Self, from spirit, one of the most reliable and effective routes back is through my body, my breath—and through conscious movement.

When you feel alive, vital, present, there's energy moving and flowing through you. This movement of energy is the essence of both health and creativity. To feel "stuck," on the other hand, is to feel no movement. It's to stiffen, to come to a standstill, a stasis. Fear itself is synonymous with non-movement, with paralysis, the inability to take action. When you're afraid, you literally become "frozen."

One of the best antidotes to fear, or the experience of being stuck, is to simply get moving again—to run, hike, walk, stretch, do yoga, dance, play. Physical activity of this kind stimulates your energy, helps you unwind internally, and opens your creative channels. New ideas and insights enter your awareness. You start to feel alive again, vibrant, optimistic. You begin to see opportunities where none existed before.

My work as a healer is fundamentally about movement—the creating of a new movement of energy. The chiropractic and related therapies I use in my office move muscles and joints, bringing the body's structure into a more optimal alignment so that the patient's physical, mental, and emotional energies can flow more cohesively. When these energies are in balance much sickness and pain disappears, and the patient feels a renewed wholeness, a more authentic sense of Self. A regular program of movement, of exercise, helps the individual maintain this new sense of well-being.

Freeing Up the Flow of Energy

Grasping the importance of movement in your life is one of the big secrets. Once you know it, then whenever you're feeling depressed, or out of sorts in any way, you have the key to shifting your energy. Stephano Sabetti, a therapist and workshop leader who taught me much about being more present in my body, often said that his entire work was about movement. "The importance of movement," he said, "is its fostering of awareness of the flow of life energy."

In his workshops he would have people breathe, flex, stretch, and do other subtle movements in order to free up a blocked, or dysfunctional, pattern of energy. By gently but persistently amplifying whatever the movement was—a sense of confusion in the head, a feeling of fear in the gut, a cry held in the throat—a change would come about.

This technique is the basis of body-oriented psychotherapies such as Reichian work, Radix, and bioenergetics. By encouraging the person to feel whatever they are feeling more fully and completely, the feeling intensifies. It builds to a peak, and is followed by a catharsis, a breakthrough into a new awareness, a new energetic experience, whether physical or emotional. Such a breakthrough is the essence of transformation.

Sabetti speaks of micromovements, subtle body movements which are healing because they bring us more in touch with the fundamental pulse—or movement—of life. "Change, or growth," he writes in his book, *The Wholeness Principle*, "is basically a natural process. The principal obstacles to this natural process are our fear of change, our illusions, our belief in the existence of one reality, and our stubbornness in letting go of old habits and ideas." All these obstacles are essentially fixed ideas and attitudes we cling to and that prevent the organic movement of something new, something fresh and creative, within us.

The Yoga of Awareness and Feeling

Movement has always been an important aspect of my workshops. I teach a kind of yoga, similar to *hatha* yoga, that I learned from Jean Klein. He, in turn, was introduced to it by a master of the Kashmir Shaivite tradition in northern India. In the Kashmir tradition of spirituality, unlike other more ascetic and world-denying traditions such as Vedanta, or certain fundamentalist Buddhist and Christian sects, the goal is to discover and live one's enlightenment in the world, using whatever object or situation the world presents to us.

Through consciously embracing and learning to master embodied existence and all its expressions—which includes art, music, work, relationships, sexuality, and the way we breathe, move, and sense ourselves in our bodies—we honor Shiva, or God, the divine Reality that is behind all creation. This is the essence of Tantra, a spiritual philosophy which, rather than turning away from the world, also uses daily existence as a path back to wholeness.

In Kashmir yoga, unlike the more well-known *hatha*, the emphasis is more on the *awareness* of movement, sensation, and feeling, and less on the finished postures themselves. The movements are done slowly and gently. There's no prescribed form. It's a spontaneous process. I guide the workshop participants through various poses that help them get more in touch with the energy behind the movement. There are frequent pauses, opportunities to feel into the deep stillness that unfolds as a result of subtle, conscious movement.

Because this form of yoga, of working with the body, is so easy, it's suitable for anyone, regardless of their age or state of health. Most people love it. Doing yoga slowly and consciously in this way frees up tight muscles, stiff joints and, especially, clears away the clutter in the mind. A new energy begins to course through the body. People experience more vitality, more aliveness. It's as if their very cells are being massaged. The yoga awakens them, quickens them, at the subtlest levels of being.

The goal of yoga is, ultimately, to be able to slow down, to come to stillness within oneself so that the practitioner can experience union with God, with the higher Self. As stated by Patanjali, who formulated the philosophy of yoga in ancient times, yoga's purpose is to: "Bring about the cessation of mental activity, so that the real Self can be experienced." It's to learn to move consciously *into* stillness and openness.

The beautiful feature about this style of yoga is that it brings people to a natural stillness in a remarkably short time. The outer movement of the yoga leads to an awareness of the inner movement, the vibration of the life force within. Usually within ten or fifteen minutes in my workshops there's a palpable silence in the room, a deep feeling of calm and serenity. We're all in a state of the highest resonance with each other. For many people, this experience of stillness—of an exquisite and totally harmonious energy—is profoundly healing.

For some, it's the first real taste they've ever had of the peace that is their essential nature. Most people still tend to objectify this peaceful state, seeing it as something outside themselves, a product of the yoga, the workshop environment, the resonance of the group. They don't yet realize that it's inherently who and what they are.

For most of us, this realization, which is the truly liberating one, doesn't come until we've been on the path a long time. Again, you have to learn to stop looking outside yourself. This means that when the energy of peace and stillness is present, you must begin to feel it inside yourself, and consciously recognize it as an aspect of your true nature.

It's similar to when a good friend looks at you and says, from the heart, "Hey, I want you to know I really care about you, and I'm here for you." When you allow yourself to fully take in this kind of communication, you get it. You know you can trust him or her. So it is with that energy of peace, of love. It, too, is letting you know, "I am always here for you. You can trust me to always be here." Just as you would turn to your friend in time of need, so you learn to trust that inner feeling of well-being.

Throughout the workshop, I'm constantly attuning myself to the movement of energy in the room, and doing whatever is necessary to keep it flowing smoothly and creatively. My job is to "hold the energy," as it's often termed. It's a lesson in the dance of Grace and will. Too much control, too much willfulness on my part—too much ego!—and nothing genuinely creative can happen. There's a sense of strain, of effort. And yet if I let go too much, if I just "allow" things to drift along without any guidance, without giving some form to our participation with each other, the experience is equally unsatisfying. I need to be very present—listening, feeling, and sensing with my whole being, in order to find the balance.

With the yoga, then, I'm able to bring people to the experience of stillness, where they can touch—or at least get a sense of—the healing energy that's always available to them. Getting a feel for moving their bodies in this way also gives them something they can take home with them. They have a practice they can either use on its own, or blend with whatever other form of movement they may do. Again, it's not the technique that counts, but the awareness with which the movements are done.

Creating Your Own Form of Movement

The principle of awareness applies to any form of movement. It's the consciousness with which you do it that's important. It doesn't matter so much what style or form of movement you prefer, the main thing is to move. For movement, as you're perhaps beginning to appreciate, releases blocked energy and creates a new sense of aliveness in both the body and the mind.

This is one of the main values of exercise. Without doubt, regular, conscious exercise is one of the best ways of keeping your creative energy moving—and ensuring, in the process, that you have a healthy relationship with your body. I've seen this time and time again in my own practice: it's the patients who have committed themselves to exercising on a regular basis, making movement an important part of their lives, who have the fewest health problems and who are generally the most mentally and emotionally stable.

Exercise is so vital that its role in everyday health can't be overemphasized. Exercise, so long as it's not carried to an extreme, is always rejuvenating. It helps your joints stay supple and flexible, ensures your heart and lungs remain healthy, and keeps your blood and your energy circulating.

There are two types of exercise, two forms of movement, that you need in order to maintain a high degree of well-being. The first is aerobic exercise, which is anything that gets you breathing more deeply and quickly, thereby increasing your heart rate. Walking, jogging, cycling, swimming, tennis, dance, and rowing are all good examples of aerobic exercise. What matters is that you find an exercise you enjoy doing, one that you can actually look forward to four or five times a week, not only for the activity itself, but because you know that you're doing yourself good by engaging in it.

The other kind of exercise you need in order to maintain a high level of physical well-being is some form of daily stretching. Flexible, open joints help prevent arthritis from developing. Gentle movement and stretching exercises keep you from getting stiff, and allow the energy to flow evenly and smoothly throughout your whole body, without the kind of blockage or interruption that manifests as stiffness, soreness, and pain.

An easy ten or fifteen minutes a day of stretching, bending, twisting, and flexing, whether in the morning or evening, is usually enough to keep your body loose and limber, especially if you're already reasonably flexible. If you're very stiff, and aren't used to stretching, you may need a somewhat longer work-out.

My own preference for stretching is, as I've indicated, yoga. I learned the basic postures from a book initially, then later took some classes in order to expand and refine my practice. Over the years, as my body relaxed and I became more supple, I found that I didn't need to do as much yoga. A few basic stretches each morning, and a longer session three or four times each week where I'd go more deeply into my favorite *asanas*, or postures, were enough to keep me feeling healthy. In fact, after many years of regular, but not especially intensive yoga, I'm now more flexible than I was when I was twenty years old.

I've seen this happen with others, as well—people in their fifties, sixties, and even older taking up yoga, and in time, regaining a suppleness and ease of being in their bodies that they assumed they'd lost forever. It's amazing how much recuperative and regenerative power our bodies have, if we'd but give them a chance.

You don't have to do yoga, of course, but it's important to commit to some form of stretching exercise, of gentle, conscious movement, to work out the stiffness and tension that inevitably accumulates in your muscles and joints. The beauty of yoga is that it's such a meditative, relaxing form of exercise. It brings about a heightened sense of well-being not only physically, but mentally, emotionally, and spiritually as well.

The Relationship between Mental Health and Physical Energy

The best exercise programs help you attain that sense of total well-being. The body, mind, and emotions are not separate from each other. They're interrelated. Each is affected by and influences the other. You may have noticed that when your body doesn't feel well, you tend to lapse more quickly into negative thinking. Similarly, when you're feeling worried, confused, angry, or upset in some way, such negative thoughts and feelings, if allowed to persist, invariably create tension and discomfort in your body. Chronically negative mental and emotional states cause enormous stress in the body. According to some estimates, they may be responsible for as much as eighty-five percent of all disease.

The value of exercise is that it creates movement in the body and in the mind. Movement brings freedom to stiff joints and tight muscles. At a subtler level, this kind of movement facilitates a healing flow of energy throughout the entire body, including our organs, glands, and the cells themselves.

This current of energy, as you're now beginning to appreciate, is felt as aliveness, vitality, radiant well-being. Learn from the example of children. They show us that movement is indeed one of the secrets of life. Children naturally enjoy a high degree of suppleness and activity. From the minute they wake up, they're almost continually in motion. Take a person who is very old and feeling his or her age, however, and you'll see the opposite—a marked lack of movement, energy, and frequently, health. Consider, for a moment, this verse from Stephen Mitchell's beautifully written version of the *Tao Te Ching*, the ancient Chinese manual on the art of harmonious living:

Men are born soft and supple;
dead, they are stiff and hard.
Plants are born tender and pliant;
dead, they are brittle and dry.

Thus, whoever is stiff and inflexible
is a disciple of death.
Whoever is soft and yielding
is a disciple of life.

The hard and stiff will be broken.
The soft and supple will prevail.

An ongoing program of exercise, of conscious movement that combines both aerobic activity and the more relaxing effects of daily stretching and flexing, will help you maintain a natural youthfulness and vitality. Such a program will support you in moving through life in a more balanced way, and enable you to experience greater harmony in body, mind, and spirit.

A conscious, healthy diet is essential for inner clarity and physical well-being.

Chapter 5
Eat for Energy

Along with exercise and movement, it's the food you eat that has the most direct effect on your energy and the quality of your awareness. Paying conscious attention to your diet will support your physical well-being while, at the same time, making it easier for you to find the mental, emotional, and spiritual harmony you're seeking.

It's been said that you are what you eat. There's a great deal of truth behind this statement. You take on the energy of the foods you ingest. Heavy foods like red meat, or any dish which is very rich or fatty, tend to make you feel heavy and, especially if you overdo it, sluggish. They use up a lot of energy in the digestive process. While they may stimulate you initially, you may find that a few hours later they leave you feeling depleted.

Lighter foods, such as grains, vegetables, and fruits put much less stress on your digestive tract. They require very little energy to digest and are so rich in vitamins, minerals, and other nutrients that they actually give you more energy. This is one of the reasons why people who follow a predominantly vegetarian diet often have a consistently higher level of energy and endurance than individuals who eat a lot of meat and other rich or concentrated foods.

Fruits, vegetables, and grains are also natural foods. This means that they are free of chemical additives, assuming they haven't been sprayed. When they break down in the digestive system, therefore, there are no harmful by-products or residues. The only effect of eating them is better health. Indeed, the foods in these groups constitute the most healing diet of all, and many people have healed themselves of degenerative diseases and other health problems through following such a diet.

Too much meat or refined or processed foodstuffs, on the other hand, can be a definite health risk. For a start, there are the chemicals—the drugs, hormones, and other additives—that are usually found within them. Most beef cattle, for instance, are fed growth hormones and antibiotic drugs. Chickens are given similar drugs, which means that the eggs you buy in the supermarket—unless they are labeled "natural, free range"—have those same drugs and hormones in them. Many individuals are highly allergic to these chemicals, and the long term risks and effects on health have been far from fully ascertained.

The role of fat and cholesterol in heart disease is common knowledge now. Less well-publicized is the fact that excessive protein consumption is a contributing factor in arthritis and other degenerative diseases. The by-products of protein metabolism, urea and uric acid, "clog" up the cellular system in the body and cause undue stress to kidney and liver function. Many individuals find their arthritic pains lessening and even disappearing altogether when they eliminate meat and dairy products from their diet. Dairy products, because of their mucous-forming tendencies, are also highly implicated in sinus problems, colds, and congestion. Cutting down on or doing away with dairy is sometimes all that is needed to restore the respiratory tract to health.

Caffeine, sugar, and alcohol also put considerable strain on the body, especially the liver, pancreas, adrenal glands, and kidneys. These refined, processed substances over-stimulate the adrenals and have an adverse effect on your blood sugar level, directly affecting the way you feel. In the short term you may find them energizing, but there is frequently a let-down in energy some hours after. If these substances are ingested in excess, the risk of a breakdown in the body's internal resources, followed by disease and debilitation, is greatly increased.

The information I have shared above is simply by way of introducing you to the importance of food, or nutrition, in health. Nutrition is a subject all by itself and there are many, many good books devoted entirely to its role in the healing of disease and the maintenance of everyday well-being. Check some of them out.

Nutrition can be a confusing issue, however, with experts in the field disagreeing with each other—often heatedly—on everything from how much protein you should eat, to the need for nutritional supplements, to the pros and cons of vegetarianism, to whether milk is good for you or not, or to the best diet for weight loss.

Finding the Best Diet for You

The best way through the confusion that's often engendered by the nutrition gurus is to begin to monitor your own dietary practices. Keeping a daily journal can be very useful. You might want to try recording everything you eat for a period of several weeks or longer. Note how what you eat affects your energy and your health. This includes how well you sleep, how you feel when you wake up in the morning, and the consistency or instability of your energy—including your mental and emotional moods—during the day. If you do this you'll discover, within a short time, definite patterns. Experiment with changing your diet, with eliminating foods or substances that have a negative effect on your energy and well-being, while adding those that support it, and youe will notice a positive difference in how you feel.

It's amazing what young people can do to themselves without apparent harm. Food, no matter how rich or excessive, usually doesn't have the same negative effect on a young person's energy as it does on someone who is older. As you age (especially when you move past your mid-thirties) you become more sensitive to foods and chemicals. It's imperative, if you want to maintain good energy and live out a healthy, full life span, that you be conscious of what you put into your body.

Diet, like exercise, is ultimately an individual matter and you'll have to experiment, as I've suggested, to find out what works best for you. As a general guideline though, natural, unprocessed foods are best. This means a diet composed chiefly of fruits, vegetables, grains, legumes, nuts, and seeds. Unless you're a total vegetarian and know your foods well, some chicken and fish will be necessary to ensure adequate protein and Vitamin B12 (which is more difficult to find in vegetable sources). You'll probably find you have a healthier respiratory and digestive tract if you cut back on dairy, and you should definitely be sparing with caffeine, sugar, and rich or spicy foods.

The simpler the diet, the easier it is for the body to handle it. Such a diet means less stress on the digestive tract, less energy taken up in digestion, more energy available for overall physical, mental, and emotional functioning. A more complex diet of heavy, rich, or spicy foods puts a greater strain on the digestive system and uses far more energy than it will give you. As with so many other areas of life, the adage to "keep it simple" applies to your dietary practices as well.

Even among advocates of "natural" health, the need for nutritional supplements is a subject of debate. It's a fact that if you eat a natural, preferably organic diet consisting mainly of vegetables, grains, and fruit, you'll almost certainly get all the vitamins and minerals your body needs. Most people are under stress, however, and even with the best of intentions, it's often difficult to consistently eat such an "ideal" diet. In this case a multi-vitamin and mineral supplement is probably of value. When you're dealing with actual disease or dysfunction in your body, specific nutritional supplementation, under the guidance of a health professional, can often be helpful.

Food and Emotional Well-Being

There's a strong relationship between emotional well-being and the food you eat. This can't be over-emphasized. Emotions, after all, are felt in the body. They are hormonal and chemical reactions that can be directly influenced by the quality of the food you ingest. Eating too much of the wrong kind of food—too much fat, too much sugar, too much carbohydrate—can lead to depression, for instance, just as surely as a negative, defeatist attitude.

People often try to drown out their negative emotions and uncomfortable feelings by overeating, by "stuffing" themselves. This can work temporarily—a kind of "pacification" effect—but if you've ever done this (and we all have!) you know there's a price to pay for such indulgence. Over-eating affects your ability to think clearly and makes you feel heavy and tired. It burdens your digestive tract. If it becomes a chronic pattern, it can result in a variety of emotional, as well as physical, problems.

The yogis in India have always had a clear understanding of the relationship between food and energy. They classify all foods as belonging to one of three categories. *Tamasic* foods, which include meat and dairy, tend to cause feelings of sluggishness and torpor. *Rajasic* foods are the stimulants and spices—for example, caffeine, ginger, garlic, onions—that accelerate the body's metabolism and can over-excite the emotions. *Sattvic* foods are fruits, vegetables, and grains. They bring harmony and balance to the system. For someone on the path of enlightenment, *tamasic* and *rajasic* foods may be used with discretion, but a *sattvic* diet leads most quickly to the clarity that is sought.

With food it must be remembered that it's not only what you eat that's important, but also the way you eat it. Food that is selected intelligently, prepared lovingly, and eaten consciously—which means chewing it well, and not eating more than is enough to satisfy hunger—has beneficial effects far beyond its mere nutrient value.

When you eat in such a way, then your food is a sacrament. You have a relationship with it. You're taking in live energy, in the form of natural foods, and you in turn are enlivened and energized. Eating consciously like this helps you feel clear and at ease within. Indeed, you may be surprised at how healing and nourishing your food can be.

You've probably found already, however, that changing your dietary habits is one of the most difficult changes of all to make! It's not like giving up alcohol and cigarettes (which is difficult enough), because these are things you can live without anyway. Indeed, you live better without them.

But you must eat, and for many of us food itself becomes an addiction which fulfills a variety of emotional and social needs, far beyond our actual nutritional requirements. If you're dealing with food as an addiction in this way, it may help to remember that once your long-term well-being becomes more important to you than any short-term emotional benefit you get from eating itself, food will cease to rule you.

You'll be guided by a vision of radiant health and energy, and this will soon become much more attractive to you than the idea of burdening your digestive tract with foods that, in the end, only detract from how you feel.

Learning to observe your own thoughts gives you some detachment from them, and brings a quality of spaciousness to your mind. It's this spaciousness that gives rise to clear, intelligent, creative thinking.

Chapter 6
Open Your Mind

The first four chapters in this book dealt with very physical, practical things. The focus has been on the art of being centered, grounded, and at ease in your body. The body-based approach is the foundation of true well-being. It's the surest way of opening to a deeper experience of your own innate wholeness.

This work with the body needs continual reinforcement. Too often, in our fast-moving, information-oriented culture, we tend to overlook it. Caught up in the daily whirl of life and all the things we feel we must think and worry about, we take our body and our physical well-being for granted. Yet without a conscious, healthy relationship with our bodies, it's a lot harder to maintain mental clarity and emotional stability. The better we feel physically, on the other hand, the clearer and more potent our thoughts, and the better we feel about ourselves.

As I suggested in Chapter Three, it's not necessary to be in excellent health to have peace of mind. Many very sick people are able to use their illness to come to a place of genuine self-acceptance and inner peace. But it makes it easier to be at peace within if you feel good in your body. This is especially so if you're still struggling with emotional conflicts and issues of self-esteem. Taking care of the physical gives you a solid, stable base from which you can then deepen your inner work.

Once you've begun to attend to your body, it's then important to start examining your mind—both *what* you think, and the *way* you think. One of my favorite teachings of the Buddha tells us that, "All the ten thousand things are created by a single thought." This is a beautiful and succinct way of saying that everything you perceive is created by your state of mind—that your experience of reality, of the conditions and circumstances in your life, results from the kinds of thoughts you have.

If, for example, you tend to think about life in a negative and pessimistic way, you'll be inclined to see things as negative and pessimistic. Even a situation that someone else, someone more positive, might consider an opportunity for growth and change, will in all likelihood appear to you as cause for further despair. You may be in a new relationship, for example, and it feels so good that you just don't trust it. "This can't last, something is bound to go wrong and I'll end up getting hurt again," you may find yourself thinking. You may have been hurt in the past, and the memory of that hurt—the past, with all its negative emotional impact—continues to run you.

The chances are you may know somebody like this—a prophet of doom—and perhaps you've even felt this way yourself at times. Most of us have. It's called being a "victim." It's the gut-wrenching feeling of always being at the effect of events and circumstances, with no power to make any kind of real or meaningful change in your life. It's both an emotional viewpoint and a way of living that leads to recurring feelings of limitation, frustration, and lack. It's a guaranteed path to unhappiness, and it's sad that so many people find themselves taking it.

Look at people who are successful in life, however, people who are creating something that is meaningful for them and who enjoy the adventure of living, and you'll find individuals who hold a much brighter view of reality. They see problems as opportunities. When faced with obstacles, they take a realistically optimistic view: "I'll find a way through this," or, "It will work out somehow." They have what very competitive people would call a winner's attitude. They focus on what they want in life, the goals they wish to achieve, and their thoughts all tend to run toward supporting the attainment of those goals.

Someone whom we might think of as a loser, on the other hand, tends to be focused on negatives, on what's wrong with a situation rather than what's right. Such people are continually distracted by what they perceive as problems and obstacles. They are forever tallying the odds that are stacked against them, such as their unhappy past, their disadvantaged circumstances, their lack of supportive friends, the fact that few opportunities come their way, and so on. In the words of the old saying, they see the glass as half-empty, never as half-full.

Negative people's thinking tends to be fragmented, ineffective, and this scatters their energy, leaving them powerless over their own lives. They have lots of reasons as to why they aren't happy, and very little in the way of positive results, or accomplishments, they can point to in their lives. Such negative thinking leads directly to mental and emotional suffering—and, very often, physical disease. Negative thinking goes against the naturally expansive, creative energy of life. It leads nowhere, other than to increasing feelings of depression and low self-esteem. As your understanding of this truth deepens, you learn naturally to leave negative thinking alone, to refuse to indulge in it. You'll realize you can't afford it. It would be like eating contaminated food. It's just too unhealthy.

Positive Thinking

The first self-help book I ever read was Norman Vincent Peale's classic, *The Power Of Positive Thinking*. I was eighteen years old at the time, and was applying for a commission in the New Zealand army. At that age, and with the consciousness I had then, no career seemed more romantic or adventurous to me than that of an army officer.

This was before I was posted to Vietnam and began to wake up to the reality of war, and to what the military was all about!

I didn't have a lot of confidence that my application was going to be accepted. The competition was tough and I had been out of school for several years. In addition to that, I had only the minimal educational requirements. I felt at a considerable disadvantage alongside the other applicants, most of whom were still high school seniors, from the upper academic echelons. For several months prior to the four-day selection course I studied Dr. Peale's book every day, and gradually began to convince myself that I *could*, indeed, pass the course if I but continued to believe that I could—and if my faith in God and in myself was strong enough.

We were to undergo a rigorous testing of our physical, mental, and social aptitudes to see whether or not we were "officer material." At times I had doubts about my own suitability. It was probably just a fear that I simply wasn't "good enough" to become an army officer, and that I'd have to go back to being a clerk in an office, or something (so it seemed to me) similarly mundane and boring.

But I clung to the positive view because so much hinged on making it into the army. It was my chance for a better life, for a life of excitement and adventure. It was my chance to be somebody, to follow a career where I would have authority, responsibility, respect. If I could just keep the faith, Dr. Peale assured me, then everything I longed for would eventually come to me.

In the end I made it through the course. There were sixteen of us who passed, out of thirty-two applicants. When the Brigadier supervising the course congratulated me on my selection, and told me that I was the "kind of chap" they were looking for (he acknowledged my less than ideal academic credentials, but said that my enthusiasm, common sense, and leadership potential more than compensated!), I was overwhelmed with gratitude. I silently poured out my thanks to both God and Dr. Peale for my good fortune.

In subsequent years, whenever I felt my confidence failing me, I'd resort to the power of positive thinking, just as I would offer a prayer to God whenever I was especially grateful for something good that had happened, or when I was in trouble and needed help. Needless to say, the power of prayer and positive thinking served me particularly well when I was in Vietnam, and faced my fear of death for the first time.

I imagine that, for new readers, especially those who are just beginning to be conscious of the ability they have to control their own destiny, *The Power Of Positive Thinking* is still a potentially life-changing book. What makes it so special, I feel, is that it's a very spiritual book. For Norman Vincent Peale, himself a minister of religion, true power comes from God. It manifests *through* us, but it comes from that larger Power—whether we call it God, the Life Force, Buddha-nature, or something else—which has created us.

As Dr. Peale points out so clearly, so much of our suffering comes directly out of our attitudes toward ourselves and toward life, from our negative thoughts, opinions, and judgments. "Attitude," I read on a poster I saw once, "is the paintbrush of the mind. It colors everything you see."

To heal yourself and find inner peace, you need to begin to look at your attitudes, and to change the way you think. You do this by first of all beginning to appreciate the true power of thought—that "what you think, you are."

Observing Your Thoughts

As you learn to pay attention to your thoughts, you can begin to catch the negative, limiting thoughts and consciously choose to replace them with more positive ones. Becoming aware of your thoughts and then making a choice around them, is one of the first steps in developing some detachment from your experience—in opening up to the "witness" faculty within you, the ability to mentally stand back, so to speak, and just observe what's passing through your mind.

Learning to witness the contents of your mind in this way is an essential step for inner freedom. When you're unable to detach yourself from your thoughts and just observe them, then you're caught up in them. You're identified with them. You're at the effect of them. They have power over you. It's this feeling of being controlled by your thoughts that is behind your emotional reactivity, and most of the suffering you experience.

As you develop this capacity to just observe, to be aware—and this is really the heart of meditation—you find yourself more in a position of *choice*. You experience a new power to actually choose what you wish to think, and how you want to use your mind. This ability to stand back, to be inwardly detached from your thoughts, creates space in your mind. In the space that opens up there is room for newer, fresher thoughts to come in, for the kind of thinking that can lead to a more positive and healing view of reality.

The Limits of Positive Thinking

There are a few things you have to be careful of, however, even as you develop this ability to exercise control over your thoughts. While positive thinking and affirmations can go a long way in helping re-orient your mind so that you feel more optimistic, and more hopeful, there are some limitations to using the power of conscious thinking in this way. All too often, positive thinking can cover up, overlay, a deeper negative thought or belief. This is especially true if you tend to be mental, or intellectual, in the way you react to and process your experience. An over-intellectualized approach to living cuts you off from what you're feeling and sensing. It doesn't allow for the expression of your deeper emotional and spiritual self.

When this is the case, all your efforts to "reprogram" yourself to have a more positive attitude can work against you. As soon as something in your environment—a person, a situation—causes an underlying negative belief or emotion to surface, it can throw you into upset. I've known many "positive" thinkers over the years (myself included) whose efforts at positive thinking merely camouflaged a deeper psychological struggle, derived from an essentially negative self-concept.

In fact, the more you persist in trying to "think" positively without an awareness and understanding of your emotional make-up, the more conflict you'll experience. It will show in the tension in your face and in your body, in the artificiality and strain of your smile, in the automatic, repetitive nature of the words you use, and in the general lack of spontaneity and creativity you exhibit in your actions and behavior.

You may notice this in certain people who work in sales, for example, especially those whose hearts are not in their work. They have so programmed themselves with affirmations and positive attitudes that there's something unnatural, almost mechanical, about them. They don't respond authentically from their hearts, but meet each situation from their rigid mental programs. There's nothing "enlightened" about this way of being at all. When doing business they tend to act like robots, motivated by one purpose only—to get the sale.

The Best Thinking Comes Out of a Quiet Mind

As I've outlined above, the weakness of the positive thinking approach is that it tends to be too mental. Obsessive thinking, whether "positive" or "negative," prevents you from opening up to subtler layers of feeling, intuition, and perception. By definition, people who use "positive thinking" as a tool want more control in their lives.

When you're too invested in controlling every thought and experience you have, you're limiting the possibility of anything really new or creative from arising. The most creative and brilliant thinking, for example, needs space, openness, receptivity, waiting. It needs quietness, emptiness, a balance of reverie and poised alertness. The ego that wants to control and think only certain thoughts has to quiet down, get out of the way, for the freshest and best thinking to occur.

Nevertheless, positive thinking can be a useful tool when you want to accomplish a desired goal or result in your life, especially when you use affirmative thoughts in conjunction with your powers of visualization and imagination. You may, for example, decide that you would like to find a new job, something more satisfying than the work you're doing now. Continually affirming to yourself a statement such as, "I know and trust that the perfect job is waiting for me," coupled with a strong visual image of what the job might look or feel like, will help create a sense of positive expectancy inside you. This will give you confidence as you search for your ideal job, and it will make you more alert to any potential opportunities that come your way. When you have this kind of positive frame of mind, there's an energy you put out which often brings to you exactly the thing you're looking for.

Positive thinking can be powerful when it comes to creating changes, desired outcomes, in the material world. It works a little differently, however, in terms of finding the inner peace and emotional fulfillment your heart longs for (and without these treasures, what satisfaction is to be had in material results?).

The greatest spiritual wisdom, both of the East and of the West, teaches us that true peace and joy only begin to unfold as we learn to get *quiet* within—as we learn to let go of our obsessive thinking and fretting, the ceaseless mental chatter that serves only to reinforce the "me," the ego. You may affirm to yourself, "I am at peace now," and such an affirmation may well help you become more quiet and relaxed within. The proof that you're at peace, however, will be when you notice that your mind has calmed down and you're no longer needing to affirm anything.

For real peace to unfold, thinking itself has to subside and make room for a new energy, or feeling to emerge. Then, in the peace that you're experiencing, your thinking will be more creative. There'll be a freshness and an originality to your thoughts. You won't have to "try" to be positive. It will happen naturally and effortlessly.

At those times when you're not at peace, however, it's always more beneficial to affirm a positive view of a situation rather than a negative one. From the perspective of aligning your creative energies towards producing a result, it's far better to say, "I can achieve what I want," rather than throw up your hands in despair and say, "I can't do it!"

If you say to yourself, "I feel awful!" or "I hate myself!" you'll just reinforce the conflict and unhappiness you feel, and almost certainly make matters worse. If, on the other hand, you accept that you feel bad, but say to yourself something like, "I know that peace is not far away, and so I shall breathe deeply, relax, and wait for peace to come," you'll notice a shift in your energy. You may need to keep affirming this quietly and insistently, but sooner or later such an attitude of mind will bring about a letting go within you. You'll start to relax, and the peace you seek will come.

Attaining Clarity

Positive thinking, then, is a powerful healing tool, but the real freedom in life, the freedom which brings about the full release of your innate healing and creative energies, lies beyond thought. This freedom comes as you get beyond the mind's endless noise and chatter, and discover the energy that gives rise to thought itself. This is where your meditation, your inner work, ultimately takes you. It doesn't just focus or clarify your mind; it *opens* it to the intelligence and power of the universe itself, to what you might call Universal Mind.

Why is it so difficult to get your mind quiet and clear so that you can open up to something new? A big part of the problem is that, if you're like most people, you probably make the mistake of thinking that you *are* your thoughts, and so consequently your thoughts tend to control you, to run you. This is why meditation is so important on the path of healing, taking time each day to just sit and be quiet, and get really still inside.

As you do this (and I'll go into the subject of meditation more fully in a later chapter), your thoughts tend to clear naturally, and you begin to awaken to a different quality of energy, to the silence out of which thoughts themselves arise. You start to sense, to feel, the wholeness and peace that is your true nature, and in this wholeness you begin to find more freedom from the bondage of thought. It starts to dawn on you that thought, the mind itself, is an *expression* of who you are—your essential Self—but it's not "who" you are. You begin to realize that you have thoughts, but you are not your thoughts—just as you have a body, but you are not your body, and you have feelings, but you are not your feelings.

For now, begin to play with the idea that you are not your thoughts, but rather you're the *awareness*, the intelligence, that's behind them. You're the consciousness in which the thinking process, in all its complexity and creativity, manifests—in which an endless variety of thoughts are continually arising and disappearing. In certain Eastern traditions this awareness that is your real nature is called the Self, Brahman, or the "witness." In liberal Christian theology it's known as the "Christ-consciousness." In Zen it's simply your Buddha-nature, your original Mind.

You are Not Your Thoughts

How have you allowed thought to take over in such a way that it can literally play havoc with your internal well-being? It's simple, really.

Thinking is a function of the mind, just as memory is. The "error" you've made (known as *avidya*, or ignorance, in Vedanta philosophy) is that you've become *identified* with your thoughts. Like all people, you have a long history of remembered experience, of beliefs, values, and emotionally-charged memories you cling to, and reinforce through constantly thinking about them. This personal history forms the basis of your psychological identity, your personality, your ego.

The irony, however, is that your personal history is not real. The events that happened to you in the past, whether pleasurable or painful, were real at the time, but they are no longer real now. Only the memory of them is real, and only then because you keep the memory alive through constantly thinking—in some cases, obsessing!—about them. And you continually ruminate on the past, of course, precisely because this sense of personal history—of being a "person" with a history, even though it may not be a very happy one—is what gives you your identity. Out of the beliefs you've formed about your past experience comes your self-image, your self-concept, your ego.

When you really look at it, you begin to see that this identity you've created through endlessly thinking about yourself and your life, is in fact a case of *mistaken* identity. After all, your thoughts and beliefs have no reality in and of themselves. How often, over the course of your life, have you let go of a belief, or an old behavior—along with the mindset that supports it—because you've seen that it's no longer valid or meaningful for you?

Yet at the time, you probably held the belief or lifestyle sacrosanct, to the degree that you may have even been prepared to fight for it; sometimes, for a political or religious belief, even die or kill for it. An obvious example of this from Biblical history is that of the apostle Paul, a pious Jew and persecutor of Christians, who underwent a conversion experience on the road to Damascus. In a blinding flash of illumination he saw the untenability, the falseness, of his previous way of thinking, and became an ardent devotee of Christ and his message of peace, love, and healing.

You need look no further than the mini-conversions you've undergone in your own life, the changing nature of your beliefs, thoughts, and goals as you've grown and matured. Very often your tastes in music, reading, hobbies, interests, even politics have undergone quite marked changes, not to mention the kind of work you may enjoy doing now, versus five or ten years ago, or the sort of people with whom you like to relate. Yet if you look at what you "believe" now and then remember how you were ten years ago, you may notice that back then you could not have imagined yourself thinking or feeling the way you do now.

To be aware of this in yourself is all the proof you need to see that thoughts—even whole systems of belief—in themselves are not real. They only appear real to the extent that you attach to them and give them energy, and thus life. You do this through such standard psychological ploys as justifying, validating, and defending your beliefs and ideas, while at the same time seeking to attack or eliminate opposing, or contradictory, points of view. You further support yourself in this by forming friendships with people who agree with your world view, while studiously avoiding those who have a different perspective.

Letting Go of Self-Concepts

If you are not your thoughts and beliefs, then what are you? If you let go of this personal history from which you've derived your sense of identity and formed your ego, what do you have to replace it with? Again, this is where the healing, or spiritual, journey ultimately leads. "I used to have a personal history," said Don Juan, Carlos Castaneda's teacher, "but then one day I found that, like smoking and drinking, it was no longer necessary, so I dropped it."

The idea of just "dropping" your personal history may not only sound difficult, but it may also be extremely threatening to you! After all, this identity you've formed for yourself, which is founded on all your memories, your beliefs, your hopes and your ideals, is what gives meaning to your life. Yet what you'll find as you open your mind and deepen your spiritual awareness, your sensitivity to the underlying creative force in life, is that this personal history you've become so attached to will just naturally begin to fall away.

As you learn to live more fully in the present, as you get more in touch with the energy of wholeness that is your spiritual nature, you'll begin to see, like Don Juan, that your personal history—and the need for self-concepts of any kind—doesn't really matter very much. It deserves to be honored at a certain relative level but, in the grand scheme of things, it's basically a soap opera, the drama of your past. As you awaken spiritually you'll find your true identity in *Being* itself—in the fullness and joy that you feel simply as a result of being alive.

This is the real healing, the real transformation, and as it takes hold in you, your thinking will naturally change. You'll no longer be so distracted by or identified with the thoughts that pass through your mind. Psychological and emotional memory will no longer have such a hold on you. You'll find yourself quickly and easily letting go of any negative thoughts that may arise, such as thoughts about lack and calamity, or sickness and disease. You'll understand how clinging to such thoughts does tend to create the conditions they symbolize, and that by freeing yourself of them, you open yourself up to the health and happiness that is your birthright.

As this transformation deepens, you'll find yourself more centered in your real nature, more established in that clarity and spaciousness that the Zen masters call "empty mind." With your new clarity you'll see thinking for what it is: a tool, an instrument of your awareness, your Beingness. You'll use thought for the powerful tool it is—analytical, logical, rational, intuitive—but you'll no longer be controlled by it. As the Indian saint Ramakrishna said, the mind makes a good servant, but a poor master. Instead of dominating and ruling you, your mind will become your ally, your friend.

There is great freedom when you have this relationship with your mind. It allows you to be both detached, and at the same time, extraordinarily present, fully sensitive, aware, receptive to feeling. Such clarity of mind enables you to see the big picture, the most pressing need, in any situation. It means you can entertain paradox, contradiction, and no longer be bothered by it. You can understand how something can seem black one moment and white the next—and how it can have both black and white in it at the same time, so that all you see are varying shades of grays! Such is the play of consciousness, the marvel and the mystery of life. When you're no longer identified with the black or the white, or the grays, then you're free to enjoy them as you choose—and respond to them appropriately.

To attain this clarity then, you must begin to observe your thoughts, and especially, notice your attachment to the things you think about. Don't try and rid yourself of thoughts. This is always a wearying, confusing, and never-ending process—and a delusionary one, besides. After all, the mind's nature is activity, movement. Your mind has been given to you for the purpose of generating the new thoughts and ideas you need to be successful in life. You don't want to turn that fountain of inspiration off, but you do want to get free of the old, tiresome psychological tape-loops that keep new energy from coming through.

Shifting Your Perspective

The secret is to learn to shift your perspective. Instead of being so identified with the thoughts that are arising within your mind, begin to practice identifying more with your real nature, with what is always present *behind* your thoughts. It's learning to get a sense of yourself as the *space*, the consciousness, in which thoughts arise.

Notice that by virtue of the fact that you *can* observe your thoughts, you cannot be what you're observing. Rather, you're whatever it is that's doing the looking. And what is looking is simply awareness—the pure, empty Awareness that you fundamentally are. The clear, innocent mind you were born with, before all the layers of thought and conditioning began to accumulate.

Start by being more present with whatever you're experiencing. Then become interested in presence itself—in the quality of your attention and sensitivity to what is—rather than the thoughts, concepts, or objects of which you may be aware. Focus on the *perceiving*, in other words, rather than on what is perceived. Pay attention to the act of *listening*, rather than to what is heard. Be the *seeing*, rather than get distracted by what is seen. Start getting used to being in *awareness* itself, rather than getting enmeshed in the thoughts and things of which you are aware.

The ability to be present like this is the essence of meditation. It means learning to be quiet and still so that you can awaken to deeper levels of perception, rather than being "hooked" by what you're perceiving. In time, as you do this, you'll find that emotionally-charged thoughts, memories, and beliefs will cease to exert such a grip on you. You'll find yourself experiencing less and less "psychological," or self-centered, thinking.

You'll take thinking—and yourself, and life—a whole lot less personally, and this is when authentic freedom begins. When you're no longer so burdened by endless rounds of self-obsession and "me" centered thinking, then your real Self can shine through. Then there's space in your mind for more creative thinking—clear, imaginative, intuitive, focused—and living itself becomes more of a dance, a rich and creative adventure.

The experience of spiritual well-being is above all a feeling. Becoming more sensitive to what you're feeling, both emotionally and at a more subtle, energetic level, opens your heart and helps you get more in touch with your true Self.

Chapter 7
Trust Your Feelings

One of the surest ways of getting out of your mind and the limitations of thought into a deeper experience of spirituality, is through opening up to your "felt" reality. It's to become attuned to the deeper realm of feelings, emotions, sensations—the subtle, yet palpable, energies that underlie words, concepts, and physical appearances.

My own awareness of feelings—especially of emotions—took a quantum leap many years ago when I attended a five-day human potential workshop which was designed to help people be more authentically themselves. On the third evening of the workshop, the instructor had us do a process in which we sat in pairs, opposite each other. One person had to ask the question, "What do you want?" while the other listened intently, searched within, and responded with whatever came up.

The lights had been turned down for this exercise and there was definitely a certain mood, or tension, in the room. Clearly, the two previous evenings had been building toward this moment. My partner took the role of questioner first. I began to speak of some of the things I thought I wanted, things that I thought would make me happy. As the exercise went on and the question penetrated more deeply into my consciousness, I became aware of a lot of noise and disturbance around me. Some people were starting to cry, to call out, to yell even. Another person was laughing. A woman on the other side of the room began wailing.

I, however, was my usual controlled self. I probably felt somewhat condescending toward those people who couldn't get a grip on themselves, and who had begun to break down. Meanwhile, I continued to delve into my own memory banks for what it was I really wanted in my life.

Then, quite unexpectedly, a clear, vivid image popped into my mind—an image I had never consciously held before. It was a picture of Briar, my wife at that time, and me. We were dancing happily through a beautiful meadow, with a young child between us, holding our hands. Something about that image stirred an unfamiliar feeling inside me, a deep yearning.

I found myself thinking of my own family, the one I'd been raised in, and how I had longed for family unity, for harmony, for love, but what had been there so much of the time was conflict. As I looked at the images coming forth, I began to feel tears well up, tears I hadn't allowed myself to feel in many, many years. As soon as they started to surface, I choked them back, stifled them. The images began to fade.

But as I listened to the pain and grief in the room around me, which had now become clamorous, an emotional free-for-all, I remembered why I'd come to this workshop. I had come to learn about myself, to open my heart. Suddenly I realized that it was okay to feel this deep sadness inside me. That was what I was there for. So I let it come. Finally, for once, I let go of my control, and I broke down. I started to cry in a way I'd never done. My whole body shook as I cried for the innocence I had lost, and the love I so desperately wanted.

The tears were enormously cleansing. They always are, I've found. Tears of sorrow have a softening effect. They melt the hardness in us; they dissolve our rigidity, they open us up to a deeper experience of ourselves. During the remaining two days of that workshop there were more tears for me—and laughter, too, a feeling of happiness, of a new emotional freedom. I couldn't put words on what was happening to me, but I knew it was good, I knew it was right.

I shall always remember how, after the workshop ended, late on Sunday evening, I went into the bathroom and happened to glance at the mirror. I saw a man grinning at me, his face and smile radiant, his blue eyes wide and alive with joy, with love. I was taken aback. Who was this beautiful human being? And then suddenly it dawned on me—it was me! I hadn't recognized myself!

It was just a few months after that workshop that Briar and I separated, and then divorced. The workshop, and others like it that came soon after, had helped each of us find more of ourselves, and one of the things we discovered was that our lives were going in different directions, and we no longer wanted to live with each other. I count it as a blessing, however, that we've always remained the best of friends.

Intellectual Understanding Gets in the Way

There was more suffering for me as I started to shut down again, to try and deny the inevitable grief and conflict I felt over the ending of our marriage. For intellectual and moral support, I read and was influenced by Ken Keyes' book, *The Handbook To Higher Consciousness*. The main theme in the book was that, as we learn to replace our addictive emotional needs with what he termed "preferences," we became freer and happier human beings.

A need was something we were convinced we couldn't live without, such as, "I need a man or woman to make me happy." A preference, on the other hand, was something we liked and wanted, but we weren't attached to having. Trying to fulfill our emotional "needs" was a sure path to suffering, according to Keyes, but if we could not get our "preferences" met, well, we still had ourselves and we could always choose—prefer—something else.

In later years I came to disagree with Keyes's approach. It made sense rationally, but it didn't work for me. I ended up using his teaching as a way of avoiding my feelings. His method was good in theory, but for me it was a mind-trap. Perhaps it was just the way I applied it, but it seemed too mental. I tried to be happy, to affirm only my preferences, but deep down I had a profound need that was being unmet.

The need, of course, was to know myself, which meant being in touch with my feelings and emotions, as well as my more impersonal spiritual Self. To cling to an intellectual schema of consciousness, no matter how "accurate" it seemed conceptually, was to simply entrench myself even more deeply in a part of me that I already knew too well—my mind. The result was that, practicing Keyes's techniques, I became more controlled than ever, and experienced an enormous amount of tension, especially in my face, where I had constructed a "mask" of happiness to hide my pain.

He Who Tastes Not, Knows Not

As Stephano Sabetti told me, when I met him some years later, "On the transformational path, everything that is false in us sooner or later falls away, and everything that is true remains." Two-and-a-half years after Briar and I separated, I met Barbara, who eventually became my second wife, and the mother of our son, Adam. Barbara, emotional powerhouse that she was, did as much as anyone in helping to loosen that mask and get me back in touch with my feelings and emotions. What was false in me, the theories, beliefs, and intellectual constructs I'd been clinging to all those years, began to fall away, and a more authentic "me" began to emerge.

The eighteen months I spent working with Stephano came at just the right time. I'd had spiritual teachers who taught me how to detach from my experience and to awaken to a more transcendent realm of Being. Now I needed someone who could help me get in touch with my emotions, so that I could be more grounded in my body, more powerful as a man—a stronger, more loving, and more creative human being.

I had a dream the very night after I met Stephano in which I was attending a workshop of his somewhere at a mountain retreat. We were taking a break, and I was writing in my journal of the wonderful things that had been opening up for me during the workshop. I was jotting down something, licking my lips with anticipation, when Stephano stepped up behind me, leaned down, and said in my ear, "You've more to taste yet."

That was a prophetic dream. With Stephano, the mask I was wearing finally cracked. During the first workshop with him I was lying on the floor on my back, breathing, feeling myself in my body, starting to get in touch with an energy within me that I knew was there, though I didn't know yet what it was. As my awareness traveled more deeply inside myself, an image floated up of my son, Adam, being born. I could see him coming down through the birth canal, struggling to get free. Something about his journey into life, and the relief that I'd felt at his having made it safely, the love I felt for him, triggered a primal impulse in me—the pain I experienced around my own birth, the sense of loss I felt as a child, the endless quest for some kind of womb-like security again.

A great cry of sadness welled up inside me. I felt my face tighten. The mask I'd worn for so many years became like porcelain. The pressure behind the mask, the pain of my suffering, grew in intensity until something had to give. I remember Stephano touching my face, bringing my attention to what was happening there. As soon as I felt his contact, the dam broke, the mask shattered into a thousand pieces, and my body was racked with an intense sobbing.

After it was all over and I lay quietly on the floor, my face felt marvelously relaxed. I felt like a newborn baby myself. Inside me there was a feeling of quiet, of peace. Much later, when I was reflecting on what I'd been through and the new sense of ease I felt, I thought of a phrase I'd read from Rumi, the Sufi poet: "He who tastes not, knows not." I remember how when I first read it I'd been struck by its truth, the deep wisdom contained within it.

Stephano had been right, and the premonitory dream had been perfect. I'd finally begun to move out of my head, away from my attachment to intellectual knowing, into a deeper experience of myself. I had begun to "taste" reality in a more authentic way.

If You Can Feel It, You Can Heal It

This is where opening up to and learning to trust your feelings takes you. You move into a fuller and richer experience of reality. The more you open up, the more you realize how empty—so often—words are. You understand how terribly barren and meaningless the intellectual life can be, especially when it doesn't flow out of something deeply felt within, when it doesn't emanate from the heart. Intellectual understanding, the ability to think logically and rationally, is an extraordinary tool. But without the heart, without feeling, it doesn't do much good at all. It can end up leading you so far from reality—your body-based experience of life—that it can both deceive you and cause you sickness and pain.

Working with Stephano helped me appreciate the beauty behind the statement that Barbara had long ago shared with me. "If you can feel it, you can heal it," she said, with that stunningly simple wisdom which was so uniquely hers. As my own experience had shown me, if you can feel your wounds, your blocked, troubled or emotionally painful areas, then you have the chance to heal them. If you ignore them or fail to notice them, then they eat away at you and can cause significant health problems. It's well-known now that many—perhaps the majority—of our illnesses and diseases are the result of emotional stress, of thwarted creativity and unacknowledged, repressed feelings.

You may not need to go through the kinds of intense experiences I went through in order to liberate your emotional self. It will depend on how much resistance you have to expressing your feelings and emotions. Generally, the greater the resistance, the more intense the catharsis when the emotional dam does finally break. Such a catharsis can happen in a workshop, it can happen in therapy, it can happen in meditation or at just about any time, if you're ready for it.

Breathing into the Feeling

The best way to deal with any strong feeling you're experiencing is to breathe into it, just as I learned to do. Deep breathing facilitates the movement of energy. As you breathe, tension may build initially, but eventually something will give, and the feeling or emotion can then move. It can have its natural expression.

With this movement something new is allowed to come into being. Following the experience of the feeling or emotion, you'll very often get insight into it. You'll have a clearer understanding of your emotional process, and it won't be just intellectual understanding. It will be understanding that comes out of personal, firsthand experience. You will, in Rumi's words, have "tasted" of something vital, something real. This is how feeling leads to healing.

Feelings are the substance of passion. They are the "juice" of life. The ability to feel deeply and be deeply sensitive to what you're feeling will enrich your life tremendously. Without that depth and sensitivity, however, living soon becomes empty. It takes on an air of futility. When you don't allow the full and natural expression of your feelings, life begins to lack meaning and purpose. To feel the joy, you must be willing to feel the pain that's there first. There's no other way. And the easiest, simplest method of allowing feelings to express themselves is to breathe into them—and just feel them, without judgment, without condemnation.

Getting Free of the Images that Cause Emotional Suffering

Getting more in touch with your feelings and emotions helps you become more sensitive to energy itself. Health, remember, is essentially a state of energy, of clear, flowing, harmonious energy. Learning to relate directly to energy at a more subtle, impersonal level—to sensation, feeling, mood, and vibration—rather than to concepts and ideas, is the key to directly accessing deeper and more nourishing states of well-being. As you become more adept at "feeling" the energy that is behind, and gives power to, words and physical phenomena, so you'll draw closer to the energy of wholeness itself, to that spiritual energy, that current of joy, which is at the heart of life.

As your sensitivity develops, for instance, you begin to see how the mind automatically tends to conceptualize feelings and emotions, giving them labels such as "fear," "anger," "sorrow," "joy," and so on. It is necessary for your emotional health to be in touch with your feelings, and to be able to identify them clearly. One of the main contributions of psychotherapy is in helping individuals learn to identify and accept their feelings. But being able to label feelings is only one level of reality, only one aspect of health. What happens when you let go of being so personally identified with these manifestations of energy that you call your feelings or emotions? What happens when you just allow whatever is there to simply be there, without any label at all, without bringing the mind, or thought, into it?

This is the point at which you start to move beyond the personal, beyond the psychological and emotional, into the transpersonal, or spiritual. It's learning to relate to your experience without the word, without having to judge, name, or label what's happening. If you're interested in awakening to a deeper spiritual well-being, then this faculty must be developed. It's to expand your awareness beyond your limited egocentric consciousness, while at the same time including your ego, so you don't deny or repress it.

With this enlarged perspective you're able to look at life more impersonally. It's really a totally different way of living—one which, as you master it, brings an increasing feeling of freedom and well-being. I invite you then to look more deeply at this subject of energy, the energy that lies beyond thoughts and concepts, beyond even emotions themselves, and see what it has to teach you, and how it can help bring you closer to your goal of true healing.

To begin, it is important to realize that the creative energy of life has its own intelligence, its own wisdom. Allowed to express itself, it will find its own balance, its own organic wholeness. You can see how this balancing process happens when you fully experience an emotion. There is a discharging of the energy, a natural cleansing and reharmonizing that takes place when you allow yourself to experience an emotion fully.

To experience something is to go through it to the very end. It's this going through it that finishes it, completes it, so that it's no longer a problem or an issue for you, at least in that moment. It'll come up again, of course, but as you learn to relate to your feelings by breathing into them and allowing them to have their expression, eventually the feelings will become less intense.

As I indicated earlier, once the experience is over, then the understanding usually comes. You're able to look back and see what happened. You have the advantage of hindsight. Rarely, however, do you understand a problem—which is essentially a confusing energy process—when you're in the middle of it. Your attempts to "understand" it usually just get in the way of your capacity to experience it.

As an example, if you allow yourself to feel the sadness that wells up every time you think of a former lover who left you, you'll cry as you feel the pain of your loss. If, after the tears have ceased, you can then begin to more objectively see the person who abandoned you, it'll help you get some perspective on that painful memory. This is where meditation can really help. Meditation allows you to look at the images and memories from the past that cause pain, without getting so caught up in them. You develop a watchful distance from them.

In the calmness that follows the storm of strong emotion, you're able to consciously work with those mental pictures that are the source of so much emotional suffering. In the case of the former lover, you may begin to see that the person left you not because there was anything wrong with you so much, but just because he or she needed to move on. They had their own suffering, their own destiny, to work out. You may also become aware of how much you had projected out onto that person, and how much you thought you needed them in order to be whole.

The truth is, spiritual work is always about coming back to your own wholeness, awakening to your inner Self. You cannot experience the fullness of your own Being so long as you're attached to the idea that you need someone else to complete you, to make you happy. Much of our emotional suffering comes from this misguided belief that we need someone—or something—to make us happy.

It's one thing to lose a friend, someone you love, and to feel the pain of that. Experiencing the pain of a loss is natural and normal. What is unnatural is clinging to the memory of the loss, so that the painful feelings keep churning over and over again, sometimes for years, as you continually replay the pictures and images in your mind. As you learn to let go of those images and memories, the feelings and emotions attached to them subside, and you start to awaken to something new. You start to tap into the fullness of your own energy. This experience helps you realize that you're indeed enough, just as you are—and always have been.

Releasing Contracted Energy

Energy, by its very nature, is always in a state of movement. To try and contain it, to resist the natural movement or impulse of the energy—the state or feeling—results in conflict, pain, suffering. Suffering is a contracted energy state, a state of holding.

You can do a simple experiment for yourself. If you clench your fist very tightly, it will probably feel good to do so. There's a sense of strength, of power, in a clenched fist. But keep clenching it. Continue clenching it even more tightly, beyond the point where it feels good. Now you'll notice that it will start to feel distinctly uncomfortable. Keep bunching your fist even tighter, until the nails themselves start to dig into your hand, and you'll begin to feel pain. The small muscles in your hand and fingers will go into spasm. After a few minutes of such holding, you'll probably find that you're not enjoying the experience at all.

Now unclench your fist, let it go. Notice how good it feels to not be holding on so tightly any more—how healing it is to allow the energy in your hand and fingers to move, to flow, to do whatever it needs to do. This little exercise shows you the value of letting go, and it also illustrates why physical movement itself is so therapeutic. As you've seen in earlier chapters, stretching, flexing, and moving your body is one of the best ways of releasing contracted or blocked energy states.

Again, my own experience with yoga is a good example of how this releasing occurs. There have been many times in the past when I'd find myself feeling contracted and ill-at-ease, and I'd shift my energy through doing some yoga postures. As I started to consciously stretch and bend, I'd notice the tension in my body and mind beginning to loosen and dissolve. After ten or fifteen minutes of yoga, my previously "stuck" energy would be moving again.

Once the energy began to move, I'd take time between postures to just sit and breathe into the delicious sense of stillness that was beginning to unfold within me. I'd connect with the deeper energy, that beautiful quality of spirit, that is always here, beneath the surface tension of life—underneath the physical, mental, and emotional contraction that is the ego's experience.

The energy itself is ultimately beyond words and descriptions. It can only be experienced as we get quiet and still within. When I do talk about it to people, I sometimes use the analogy of good wine. Cheap wine, or "plonk," as we used to call it in New Zealand, where I grew up, has a very coarse energy vibration. It is thick, sweet, cloying. It's an assault on the palate and hits the stomach with a crude jolt, leaving an unpleasant aftertaste and usually an annoying headache along with it.

Much of the time, the ego's experience is like this. When you live too much from your ego, the pervasive sense of "me" and "mine," there's a tension that's always present, a feeling of chronic dissatisfaction, a sense of pressure, of being always somewhat at the effect of life's circumstances. The ego's life is basically one of conflict. Like cheap wine, it's very unfulfilling, and inevitably leaves you feeling empty.

A fine wine, however, is something else altogether. It's vibration is so pure, so clear, that you really have to be totally present with it in order to appreciate it, otherwise you'll miss its bouquet, the treasure it has to offer. It pleases the nose and dances lightly on the palate. It has a delicate smoothness, a harmony to it, and it leaves no aftermath, no dross. Indeed, with a really good wine (provided it's consumed in moderation!), the mind is made lucid and sparkling.

Such is the energy of spirit. It's like the finest wine. It's the calm that is always here, at the center of the storms and upsets whirling around you, if you'd but get quiet enough to allow its presence to be felt. However, to get to the gold that is buried deep beneath the earth—if I may use a different metaphor—you have to dig through the rock and dirt first. Before you can come upon the pure energy of spirit, of your real nature, you have to face the energies that are here—the tensions, the conflicts, the emotions, the distractions. You have to deal with your ego, the "me" that never has enough and is always clamoring for more.

Learning to Handle Intensity

The key to accessing deeper states of consciousness is learning to first be with the energy as it is. It's giving space for whatever is there to just be there, so that the muddied waters of your mind can begin to settle, allowing a deeper clarity to emerge. In this way the discordant personal energies that keep you ego-bound, trapped in your mind, are permitted to untangle. Allowing energy to move through you is not always easy, however. When the movement is very powerful, as with a strong feeling or emotion, it can bring up fear. This happened in my work with Stephano, especially when I began to encounter my anger, the rage (to do with my unresolved father/power issues) that was hidden deep within, behind the "nice guy" mask that I wore.

Dealing with intense energies can be frightening for many people, and anger is an intense energy. Relating to emotions as energy teaches you to handle greater and greater levels of intensity. You learn to experience your feelings and emotions as qualities of movement, sensation, vibration, rather than conceptualizing them as "anger," "fear," "pain" or whatever. When you conceptualize or label a feeling, you either distance yourself from it—and thus avoid really feeling it—or you reinforce it, and risk making it into something more than it is.

The key is to breathe into the pure energy of the feeling or emotion. This is how you learn to confront and stay with the deeper impulses and stirrings, the darker forces, within you, and not deny or run from them. It requires a lot of trust to do this. You have to learn to trust yourself, to trust your own inner knowing and your ability to remain present with whatever may come your way.

The resistance to the natural movement of energy originates in your mind—in the attitudes, beliefs, and ideas you cling to about what "should" be, or "ought" to be. These ideas and assumptions prevent an authentic expression from arising. It's this thwarted movement, the energy that's prevented from moving organically, that expresses itself in disease and other morbid states. Chronic emotional disturbances and such personality imbalances as being too passive and open to other people's negative energy, or too rigid and controlled, and therefore unable to accept anything new or different, are examples of dysfunctional energy patterns.

To awaken to a deeper spiritual well-being involves looking at the conceptual reality you've created in your mind, and seeing to what extent it denies or permits real aliveness and self-expression. It means observing and learning from your inner process, your judgments and beliefs, the way in which your ego attempts to control or limit your experience. All your mental constructs have to be seen and let go of so that something new can unfold within you.

As the letting go occurs, it can be extremely unsettling, for it shakes your entire foundation of reality. The awakening energy, which is felt in the body as new and powerful feelings, and in the mind as confusion, doubt, uncertainty—as well as a growing excitement at the realization of new possibilities—literally begins to break up your old constructs and ideas about who you are and what is real.

In spiritual language, this is the "dark night of the soul." When you've tasted, in moments, the fullness and joy that is your real nature, it's painful to fall back into the old, contracted patterns again. Yet the ego persists in clinging to what it knows because of the sense of security it gets, illusory though it may be. It fears its own annihilation. Sometimes the "dark night" phase can go on for years, or keep returning in different forms, as you clutch at these old attitudes and ways of being—even though you know, at some level, that they no longer work for you.

At this stage of the process of opening to energy, grounding becomes very important. This means being in your body, having both feet planted firmly on the ground. You must be centered, present for what is happening, not succumbing to the temptation to "space out" or be carried away by the energies moving through you. It's this kind of heightened but very grounded awareness that enables you to integrate the new energies.

Without this groundedness you risk becoming hypersensitive, and then it's difficult to live and function in the world without absorbing a host of negative influences, and getting sick as a result.

Feelings Come in Waves

Anxiety, insecurity, emptiness, loneliness, despair, and a wide range of vague physical problems—"weird" energies and other disturbances which have no clearly defined symptomatic pattern—are some of the many states you may encounter as you let go of old ways of being and open up to the new.

What's important to remember is that these are just states. Like all states, they will pass. When they are present, you deal with them as best you can, breathing into whatever is happening and trusting the outcome. Notice, too, how feelings and energy states come in waves. When you're grieving, for example, the grief may be intense and painful at first, but as you allow yourself to experience your sorrow, it gradually subsides and gives way to a feeling of quiet, of release, of calm.

And then, some time later, the grief, just like a wave, surges forth again—usually triggered by an image, a memory. The second, third, or fourth wave may be more intense yet, until the feeling peaks—hours, days, weeks, or months later, depending on how willing you are to embrace your experience—and the waves subside once more. Gradually, the feeling begins to lose its intensity, its hold over you. The waves of emotion become quieter, weaker, and less frequent, and the periods of calm between them get longer and longer.

The more you allow the waves to come, whatever their emotional nature, the sooner you'll get to the calm. And the calm, you'll discover, is not merely a pause, a break in the turbulent sea of emotion. Rather, it's the true condition that underlies all the changing states and feelings. It is awareness itself, the pure and luminous ground of Being, what the yogis call the timeless and ever-tranquil "substratum of existence."

In ordinary, everyday language, it's the flowing and harmonious sense of peace and connectedness you feel when your body is quiet, your mind is clear, and you're simply alert and at ease in the present moment. Viewed from this perspective, the "dark night" of intense feelings and emotions, of personal uncertainty, confusion, and despair, is seen for what it is—a passage, a testing period that you must pass through in order to come upon the deeper richness within you.

Just as the strongest steel is forged slowly, in a hot fire, so a strong character is built through the willingness to embrace the totality of whatever you're experiencing.

The Wisdom of Ignorance

One of the ways in which you may block or slow down your innate drive toward self-actualization, is the tendency you may have to always want to do something, to make something happen before its time. This impulse comes out of a lack of trust. Many people feel they must control everything, and that nothing good can happen unless they somehow make it happen.

This is one of the principal illusions of the ego, the personal self. The fact is that the innate intelligence of life—the wisdom of your authentic Self—knows what is good for you far better than your ego, your personal self with all its fears and insecurities. The peace, love, and joy you seek do not come through anything that the mind creates. They are qualities of the heart. They are expansive, healing energies that move through you, naturally and spontaneously, when you get your conceptual mind, with all its judgments and considerations, out of the way.

As you learn to stop thinking so much and just allow things to happen in their own intuitive, organic way, a healing takes place. You're allowing yourself to be in your natural state of wonder. You're just open to the moment, receptive to what is. You're alive and aware in the present. In this awareness, new inspiration will come to you, new insights, new learning. New energies can awaken. Something deeper can begin to move.

Your work, you begin to realize, is to get out of the way of the natural movement of energy and intelligence, and to simply be with it, to learn to flow with it in a state of alert, sensitive presence. To do this your analytical, conceptual mind—the "me" with all its desires and attachments—has to be out of the way.

This is the wisdom of ignorance, of an innocent mind. You see it in emotionally healthy children. Their minds are still relatively unconditioned. They haven't yet developed a dominating ego. They are open to the fullness and wonder of life in the present. They are extremely sensitive, and feel everything very deeply.

Living with Heightened Awareness

The secret is to *feel* your reality, rather than think about it. It's a matter of learning to be very sensitive to whatever is happening in the moment. It's having all your sensory radar operating, so to speak, so that you're present with your body, heart, and mind. This is done not with a view to being defensive, but because you want to learn. You want to be able to respond in the most intelligent way possible to what is *actually* happening in your environment, rather than what your mind may assume is happening.

How does this sensitivity come about? How does it look in actual practice? This is meditation in action, and you'll get more understanding of this in the chapters that follow. But it begins with learning to be still, to really open up to your inner and outer environment. It's noticing the energy, the feelings and sensations, in your body. It's being watchful of the thoughts passing through your mind. It's being aware of your posture, how your body feels to you in the space you occupy as you sit, or move through as you walk.

It's observing, becoming very aware of your surroundings, the look and feel of the room you're in, for instance. You begin by observing what is most evident, such as the design, the layout, the decor, and then you move to the subtler aspects, to the feeling, the mood, the ambience.

Outdoors, it's the same process. It's being keenly sensitive to all you perceive. You visually embrace the sky, the clouds, the hills, the trees, the buildings, the grass, the ground beneath your feet. You pay attention to the road, the stream beside you, whatever is there. You look at it all, take it all in. You open yourself up to nature, to the living quality of all that's around you, which means the animals too, and the birds. Then you listen and feel for the deeper energy, the harmony, that underlies and permeates it all.

As you become attuned to this underlying energy, you start to access a power that is much greater than any kind of power the ego can assert. It's the power of the life force itself, moving and expressing through you. You experience it in the form of intuition, inspiration, trust, and confidence. The less you rely on concepts and beliefs, the more that power becomes available to you. Watch a charismatic speaker or good group leader at work—or an accomplished artist or musician—and you'll see this kind of power in operation. Such people may use a conceptual framework, a technique, but they don't rely upon it. Rather, they know that the real creative inspiration comes out of the energy of the moment itself.

It requires discipline to be attuned in this way. Awareness is an art. What I'm talking about here is the refining of your awareness, your ability to be present, to be open and sensitive to the hidden reality behind "reality." Then you must learn to trust what you're experiencing. See the limitation of thoughts and concepts, and place your trust instead in what you're sensing and feeling.

Do this, and you'll start to get in touch with the heart of life, with the source of existence itself. You'll discover that the exquisite current of energy you feel around you is also within you, that there's only one movement. Living then starts to become rich in possibility. It's in this richness, in the felt sense of the timeless beauty and creativity of life, that you touch the ground of all healing.

You know you're healing when your happiness depends less and less on what happened in the past, or what may develop in the future, and comes more and more from the simple joy of being aware and alive in the present.

Chapter 8
Live in the Present

In a very real sense, the "now" moment is all there is. The past is an illusion, existing only in memory, and the future is yet to be, and offers few if any guarantees.

To begin to see this, to come to terms with it so that you let go of any attachment to the past and the future, and instead live your life one day at a time, one step at a time, is enormously freeing. It frees you to discover the depth, the creative potential, that exists in each moment.

The more fully you're able to "be here now" in this way, to be present with your whole being, your total awareness, the richer your experience of reality. You begin to uncover for yourself the truth behind the ageless spiritual teaching, that "everything you seek is within you and around you."

As you master the art of living in the present—of "present-time consciousness," as some call it—the past and the future come into their right perspective. Everything you've learned in the past, all the knowledge you've acquired, is available to you should you need it, but you're not psychologically or emotionally bound by it. Similarly, you can visualize and make such plans for the future as are necessary or appropriate, but you're no longer seduced by false hopes, idle daydreams, or wishful thinking. Once you know your destination, your goal, you can let it go—put it at the back of your mind, so to speak—and relish the journey.

Many of the practices that come out of the various spiritual traditions, both of the East and the West, are designed to help us live more fully in the present. As you've seen in earlier chapters, conscious breathing and the developing of a more sensitive relationship with your body is a very effective method for bringing you into the here-and-now. The work we've just explored in the preceding chapter, dealing with the art of becoming more attuned to subtle energies, to the quality of presence or vibration that is behind feelings, emotions, and physical manifestation, is another potent door to present-time consciousness.

Attachment to the Past or Future Causes Suffering

Learning to live in the present is important for a simple reason: the healing you seek—peace of mind, love, joy—is to be found only in the present, not in some remembered past or imagined future. You are either experiencing peace now, or you're not. True, the memory of something pleasant, or the anticipation of an event in the future, can stimulate a desirable feeling state, but the feeling itself is felt in the present. It exists in the here-and-now, in real time, even though the cause behind it may be imagined and therefore unreal.

There's nothing wrong with deriving pleasure from thinking about the past, or from looking forward to something good that may come about in the future. But if you depend upon these stimuli for your well-being, you may be in for an upset or disappointment. In fact, if you're like most adult human beings, you'll already have had considerable personal experience with loss, and the pain and suffering that comes with it. As a consequence, it won't surprise you to realize just how tenuous and unreliable mental states—memories of the past and thoughts about the future—are as a source of security and happiness.

Coming to this realization is a great awakening. You'll notice that it usually happens in degrees. As you grow and mature, and suffer more of the disillusion, the inevitable losses and disappointments that are an inherent aspect of life, you begin to learn something about the pain of holding on, and the unburdening that happens when you're able to let go. After all, the losses you're likely to face during the course of your life are legion: the going away of a friend, the death of a loved one, financial setback, illness, divorce, a failure or rejection of some kind, an unfulfilled dream or expectation. However big or small, these losses hurt. They cause suffering.

What this kind of suffering inevitably teaches you—if you're open to the lesson—is that whenever your mental, emotional, and spiritual well-being depends upon someone or something outside yourself, that well-being is conditional. It can never truly be yours. It's always contingent upon circumstances—and the one constant about circumstances is that, sooner or later, they will change.

Much of the wisdom handed down by the great spiritual traditions is built directly on this realization. Jesus pointed out that the kingdom of heaven is within us, and advised us to take no thought of tomorrow. Look not to the things of the world for your comfort, he taught, but rather seek the inner treasure—the spiritual kingdom within—and everything else you need will come to you.

The Buddha was born a wealthy prince, and while growing up, was sheltered from the misery, sorrow, and despair that was the lot of the common people of his day. But when he finally saw this suffering for himself, it opened his eyes to reality. Thus began his journey toward spiritual awakening, to the discovery of the truth that impermanence, or change, is the way of life. Once we realize this, the Buddha taught, then we learn not to cling to that which is inevitably going to change. Only in this approach, where there is no attachment and therefore no resistance to change, is there the possibility of true peace and happiness.

The deeper healing that you seek within yourself, and in your life, begins to take place as you come to terms with this art of living in the present. It's having the ability to let go of thoughts about the past and the future, and instead get involved and interested in where you are now, in what is happening in your life now. The themes and ideas presented in preceding chapters in this book are all designed to help you do this more effectively, and the ones that follow will give you even more tools to work with as you refine your own present-time consciousness.

Presence is Something You Can Feel

Living in the present starts with being aware of your breathing, your body, your feelings. It's being grounded in the reality of the moment, in your actual physical experience of the moment. It's being connected to your environment. If you're with other people, it's really being *with* them, being open to them, giving them your total attention. If you're engaged in an activity of some kind, it's being fully there with whatever you're doing. It's being present with *all* your energy.

You can always tell how present someone is. You know whether they're listening to you or not, whether they're distracted or not, whether they're interested or not. Presence is something you can feel. You just intuitively sense it. The contact is there, or it's not. The connection is there, or it's not. Similarly, when you have someone's attention, when you're really communicating with each other, attentively listening and sharing, you can tell when the contact is broken. You notice it immediately. It's literally as if a thread is broken, as if something is pulled away from you.

Perhaps more than any other factor, it's this ability to simply be present that opens up the way for healing to occur. Presence is awareness, attention, sensitivity. It's unconditional love. When you're just present—with a friend, with yourself, with the moment—then you're tapping into a deeper energy, into something larger than yourself, your own ideas and concepts. You're making yourself more available to the moment, with all its potential for something new.

The most enlightened people I've been around all had this quality of presence. I think especially of my spiritual teachers and others I've known. These people lived in the world with a sense of balance and harmony. They expressed that inner richness which comes with true peace of mind. They demonstrated a creative playfulness in the way they dealt with the challenges of daily living.

There was a simplicity and an ease of being about them. There was no pretense. They were not hiding behind their reputation or their credentials. They had no need to impress or convince anyone of their truth, nor were they trying to control the outcome of events. They were just being themselves, and it was their very openness, their vulnerability—not to mention their wisdom, compassion, and humility—that was the source of their power. Around them things *did* happen, and what happened always seemed to be just what was needed in that moment.

When you're able to be unconditionally present like this, you're guided by a deeper wisdom. It's not a conscious wisdom, either. It doesn't involve thought or premeditation. It just happens, a spontaneous knowing. The answers, the inspiration, the next step to take—everything is right there just when you need it. When you're present like this you're connected to the source of creativity, to the pulse and breath of life itself.

When you feel this connectedness, there's little or no sense of duality with it. You don't feel separate from what you're experiencing. There isn't "you" and "the source," or "the energy." There isn't "you" and an idea of "God," "Buddha," or some other power outside you. There's just the wholeness of life, the flow of being, and you're one with it. It's a continuum, an endless cycle of death and rebirth, of the old giving way to the new.

Throughout it all, you're simply *here*, living your life and dancing with the great mystery of existence. In Zen, the mystery is called the "suchness" of things—and you, in your essence, are as much a part of the "suchness" as the trees, the birds, the flowers, the very air you breathe.

It Requires Trust, Vulnerability, and Strength

It takes trust to have this kind of presence, this openness to and oneness with life, which is why it takes most of us a long time to come to it. It's easy to be present when you're doing something you love to do, but what if you don't know who you are and what you really want in your life? What if you're faced with something scary, something that makes you want to run in the opposite direction? Or what if you're dealing with something or someone you find boring, not worthy of your interest?

When you're truly present with your experience, boredom can't exist, for boredom is a mental state. It's the result of having certain expectations, prejudices, or attitudes which have caused you to withdraw your attention from the moment at hand. When your attention is not in the present, you can't see what the moment has to offer you. You can't expect to find any richness or joy in a situation if you're not willing to look for it. The potential in any given moment is always there, but it's not necessarily self-evident. Sometimes it has to be invited, coaxed, drawn out.

To be present requires vulnerability, receptivity, openness. It also needs strength. You've got to be able to let down your defenses, let go of your judgments, your assumptions, your expectations. To do this you have to trust yourself to be able to handle any situation that might arise, and this is where inner strength becomes necessary.

In fact the only way you really develop—or discover—inner strength is through learning to face intensity, whether it be intense joy and pleasure, or intense pain and hardship. Whenever you find yourself being challenged by a particular circumstance, life is in effect asking you to be present. Every time you meet and master such a challenge, you learn more about the art of presence itself.

Life might be inviting you to open up to a new person, a new direction, a new honesty with yourself, a new way of being. The more present you're able to be, the more certainty there is of something creative occurring. It's being willing to move beyond your old boundaries, old forms, the safety of the familiar and the secure, into an unknown dimension. As I read once, a ship is safe in a harbor, but that's not what a ship is designed for. By the same token, you weren't put here to hide out. You're here to find out who you are, and what's possible for you.

Letting go is always a risk, yes, but if you look back at the emotional risks you've already taken in your life, you'll probably notice that you've gained more than you ever gave up. You've gained in aliveness. You've grown in wisdom. You've discovered more of your true Self, your spirit, your inner resources.

Being Present with Yourself

Vulnerability and strength give balance to presence. There'll be times when you may find yourself feeling vulnerable, sensitive, and your presence may have a hesitancy to it. At such times you can be more easily hurt and will almost certainly absorb any negative energies that are around. At other times you may feel strong, confident, present to the degree that others may experience you as being somewhat heavy-handed, even invasive.

The more you know yourself through observing the different aspects of your personality, the more you can be aware of these tendencies and so come to a balance point. There can be a fine line between having no boundaries and too many, between being too flexible and too rigid, between being wishy-washy and over-bearing. It's all too easy, for many people, to tip from one end of the spectrum to the other, and all the while miss the center, where authentic presence is to be found. Life will give you feedback as to how you're doing, but in the end you have to rely on your innate sense of what feels right to tell you when you've reached that balance.

Again, the simple techniques of remembering to breathe deeply, to focus your attention on what's before you, to listen carefully, to unlock your knees if you're standing, or to have your spine straight if you're sitting, all help you to be more present. When you are in your body, when your posture and your senses are alert, you are naturally in a state of presence.

It's a state that at first can be difficult to attain, but in time, if you're genuinely seeking a deeper joy and vitality in your life, you'll realize how unsatisfying it is to not be present. Eventually you'll come to understand that what you're looking for is here now, and always has been. The more attention and sensitivity you can bring to the moment, the more alive and interesting the moment is.

Ultimately you must learn to be present with yourself. The more deeply you feel and understand yourself, the easier it is to merge with the moment. As you'll see in the next chapter, this is where meditation comes in—taking the time each day to sit and be with yourself. It's when you're able to just sit in open, alert awareness, without needing to think or do anything, that you get to know yourself. As the layers of your mental and emotional conditioning begin to rise up and peel away, so your awareness penetrates through to something deeper, to the timeless current of energy that is always here, beneath the activity of memory, thought, sensation.

That energy, you'll learn, is the very heart of presence. It's the source of thought, of all creative power. The more attuned to it you are, the more you bring its power to every moment, and every situation. Presence is within you. It's your natural state of being. In those moments when you're in your natural state of ease, living in the present isn't a problem. You're just doing it.

The work is to remember to come back to yourself, to continually come back to the present, to that quality of presence within and around you. It's a simple art, and yet it's the most elusive. It's something you need to remind yourself of again and again.

Meditation is at the heart of spiritual practice. It's through meditation that you get to know yourself at the deepest levels, and begin to come upon the inner well-being—that abiding sense of peace and contentment—that is life's richest blessing.

Chapter 9
Meditate!

For me, meditation has been the most consistent and most essential element of all the inner work I've done.

It was through meditation, through learning to sit and be with myself on a regular, daily basis, that I gradually began to find the inner stability I'd been seeking all my life. Everything else I've explored, such as yoga, psychotherapy, the dance of interpersonal relationships, and the challenge of business and being in the world, has been important, but it is meditation, the foundational practice, that has tied it all together.

Finding time to just "sit and be," whether for fifteen minutes or longer, whether once a day or twice, is the most common complaint voiced by people interested in meditation. Everybody is so busy these days. To exclaim, "I've got too much to do! I have to keep moving if ever I'm to get ahead!" seems legitimate enough. Yet the fact is you have to make time if you want to discover the healing benefits of meditation. And if you're so concerned with getting ahead, you might find it worthwhile to sit down for a bit—meditate!—and ask yourself, "Exactly where do I think I'm heading?"

Making time for meditation inevitably involves a sacrifice of some kind, though as you grow into meditation and get to like it, you won't think of it as a sacrifice at all. If you're like most people, it'll be that extra twenty or thirty minutes in bed in the morning that you'll choose to give up. The early morning is traditionally the best time to meditate anyway. Once you're fully awake your mind is generally clearest and at its most receptive, and the morning energy itself—its stillness—invites a deepening of awareness, a more effortless communion with spirit.

The second most common complaint has to do with the restlessness that many people experience when they sit to meditate. How do you deal with the noisy mind, the constant ferment of thoughts and images, of impulses and desires? How do you get beyond the mental conflicts and disturbances so that some of the joys of meditation can at last begin to be realized?

When I first began to meditate, many years ago now, it was extremely difficult for me to sit still for twenty minutes at a time and inwardly say the *mantra*, the sacred sound, that had been given me by my meditation instructor. I was by nature restless and easily bored. But the *mantra* helped. It gave a focus to my thoughts, something on which to concentrate my attention, and that brought about a degree of inner quiet. Eventually I began to experience moments of real peace and clarity. Following my meditation, I would often feel a glowing sense of well-being.

After six months I felt the *mantra* was limiting me, and I shifted more to a Zen, or *vipassana* form of meditation (*vipassana*, which means "insight," or "clear-seeing," is a Buddhist meditation practice and is similar, in some ways, to the Zen form, where you basically just sit and be present). With this new approach, I'd observe my thoughts, feelings, and body sensations as they arose, without judging them or identifying with them. This free-form style of meditation seemed more flowing and spontaneous to me. I would sit until I either felt myself becoming inwardly clear and peaceful, or until my restlessness won out and I just couldn't stand it any more!

Beginner's Mind

The person who taught me the most about meditation was J. Krishnamurti. Krishnamurti, who was internationally famous as a philosopher and spiritual teacher, once defined meditation as, simply, "The ending of thought." By this he meant that it's only when our habitual patterns of thinking, the mental and emotional "tapes" we tend to play over and over again drop away, that something new—a deeper level of insight or feeling—can come through.

This is similar to the Zen teaching of "beginner's mind." Suzuki Roshi, the Japanese Zen master who founded the San Francisco Zen Center, taught that, "In the beginner's mind, there are many possibilities; in the expert's, few." This is a beautiful statement about both meditation and the nature of enlightenment. It helps explain Jesus' teaching that you must be as a child before you can enter the kingdom of God. It's only through an open, innocent mind, a mind free of prejudice and conditioning, that you can receive God's grace—or in Zen terminology, experience your Buddha mind, your natural, awakened state of consciousness.

Through meditation, you gradually empty your mind of all your psychological and emotional programming—your opinions, beliefs, judgments, all the mental "baggage" you've accumulated over the years. In this emptying, a new clarity and freshness starts to be felt. You're wiping the slate clean of all the dross and dirt, and getting back to something original, something pure, something pristine. You're putting yourself in an open, receptive state, just like a child.

But you don't lose what's important. All the useful technical and survival knowledge you've learned about life is still there in your memory banks, available to you whenever you need it. In fact, the more you're able to be in "beginner's mind," the more access you have to this information. You don't have so much psychological "garbage"—the clutter of ego-based thinking—in the way.

Bringing Your Awareness Back to the Present

I began to explore these ideas—and especially the teachings of Krishnamurti—in my own meditation. I'd carefully watch myself inwardly, observing what I was thinking, and I'd experiment with just letting the thoughts fall away, with negating thought, as Krishnamurti called it.

Normally when a thought arises it takes you off somewhere. It literally carries you away into other realms of thought, memory, speculation—the yammer-yammer that is the mind's addiction! Then at some point, something in the present grabs your attention again—a breeze, the chirp of a bird, a shifting sensation in your body, the sound of your breathing—and you notice that you've been "off" somewhere in your head. It's this realization that you've been inattentive that brings you back to the present.

Surprisingly, it wasn't so hard to let go of the activity in my mind. I'd be sitting meditating, and a thought would float up—about a problem I was dealing with, for example. I'd just let it go, and simply come back to being aware. A moment later, I'd find myself getting lost in thought again, carried away by yet another musing coming out of seemingly nowhere. Perhaps I'd find myself thinking about a trip I was planning, a letter I needed to write, a person I'd just met—or how well my meditation was going! Then I'd come back again.

As Krishnamurti used to point out, it's unrealistic to expect to be fully aware every waking moment of the day, but you can notice when you're not being aware. And it's that awareness, the awareness of inattention—"Oops, I've been drifting off again"—that brings you back to a state of alert presence.

It's the same as when you're in conversation with a friend and you notice their attention is wandering, and you ask them to "come back," or you do something else to gently pull in their attention. In meditation, you're learning to be your own friend. It doesn't matter if you go away, or "space out." The trick is to notice you're doing it, to be aware that you're getting distracted by some train of thought or other, and then simply return to the now moment, without any fuss or self-recrimination.

A Quiet Mind Brings Clarity and Insight

Something that helped me with this process was an agreement I liked to make with myself. If I was being bothered by a problem that I was reluctant to let go of because my mind had decided it was overwhelmingly important, I'd agree to put it aside just for the fifteen minutes or so of my meditation. Later, I told myself, I could pick it up again and become as obsessed with it as I liked.

This approach helped me forget my problems temporarily, and opened up space for something fresh to come into my awareness—often a solution to the very conflict I had been grappling with. It also helped me see how artificial so many of my so-called "problems" were. All too often they were just creations of my busy, restless mind. It seemed that I got a lot of energy out of my internal conflicts—they gave a certain kind of "meaning," a quality of drama, to my life—but it wasn't a very satisfying energy.

As Krishnamurti frequently said, the perception of truth brings its own action. When you finally see that it's the incessant whirl of thoughts and images in your mind that keeps you out of the present moment, you begin to do something about what you see. You stop giving so much importance, so much energy, to your inner dialogue, to your different beliefs, expectations, judgments, comparisons. Then, in the space that opens up, you can discover something new.

I feel that all authentic traditions of meditation bring us to the same place that Krishnamurti was talking about, the place where our mind is clear and open, free of extraneous thought, and we're simply present with our awareness, our attention, our love. It's a place of stillness and silence, but it's a stillness that is dynamic, vibrantly alive.

Thoughts can arise and words can be spoken in this silence, but they don't disturb it. They are like birds flying across the sky. They appear in our vision, convey something of their beauty, their mystery, their message, and then they disappear back into the emptiness from which they came. The vast, open sky remains—the luminously clear background to all that is. In such a mind, thoughts and images, like birds winging their way overhead, leave no mark.

When you arrive at this place—and it happens for brief moments in the beginning, and then more frequently and for longer—something deeper begins to reveal itself to you. You become aware of an extraordinarily rich and full sense of being, of unity or oneness with life. Each time you touch this fullness, you experience healing and renewal. You get a new perspective on the problems and issues in your life.

Once you feel yourself to be in that very clear, expansive space you can actually invite a problem into it, an issue you may currently be working with. You might use this time of clarity and detachment to scan your life, your present situation and circumstances, to see if there's anything that needs attention.

Simply by allowing the problem to be there, and being receptive to guidance, you'll get the answers you need—if not in this sitting, then perhaps in the next one. And the guidance will come in the form of an intuition, a feeling, an image, a vision, a compelling thought or idea. Or maybe it will come in a dream one night. It's in these ways that your higher Self communicates with you.

Dealing with Restlessness and Anxiety

The challenge in meditation is to stay present with whatever you're experiencing—which, in the beginning, may well mean facing restlessness, loneliness, emptiness, anxiety. It means being willing to go through the darkness, the negativity that so often arises during the early stages of meditation. In order to grow, you're going to have to face all this anyway—the disowned aspects of yourself—and meditation is really a way of meeting it head on.

The more strongly and fully you feel yourself in your body, in contact with your physical environment, the less hold your thoughts will have on you, and the less you'll be affected by any negative or upsetting energies. Your awareness shifts out of your head into your heart, into your physicality, into the true center of your Being.

Again, conscious breathing helps with this process immensely, which is why watching or counting the breath is one of the most frequently recommended techniques for meditation. It helps too if you're able to sit comfortably, with good posture. One of the best ways of facilitating this is yoga or some other form of exercise that enhances body awareness and sensitivity.

As your awareness becomes more grounded in this way, your relationship with your mind, with thought, undergoes a major shift. You stop being controlled by the endless flow of thoughts and images, of memories and impulses. You experience more freedom from your mind, your ego. There's more clarity, more inner space. Thinking itself becomes more coherent, focused, creative. The possibility for a truly healing use of your mind, of your powers of thought, becomes a reality as you learn to master the art of meditation.

Beginning Your Meditation Practice

If you're new to meditation, here's a simple way of getting started. If you already have some experience, or are wanting to go deeper, the tips I'm sharing here might be useful for you.

The first thing to do is to find a congenial place to park your body. A place that is quiet, that is aesthetically pleasing to you, and that has a nurturing, calming feel to it, is best. It may be a room in your house where you have a view of some kind—whether of the sky, of trees, of hills, or of your garden. It's good to have living plants, or fresh flowers, in the room. You may have some objects that are spiritually meaningful to you—a picture of a religious figure, a statue, a symbol of some kind. You may light a candle. You may want to burn some incense.

I used to observe more rituals when I was new to meditation, just as I used to practice certain techniques to help me get quiet and still within. Rituals and techniques are like training wheels. They help you grow into a new way of being without getting lost or confused along the way. As it becomes easier and more natural for you to sit and attune to silence, you may find techniques and rituals an impediment. You may still like a simple ritual, but you won't let it dilute the feeling of openness and spaciousness that is the mark of true meditation.

A good length of time to allow for meditation in the beginning is fifteen to twenty minutes. As it becomes easier for you to just sit and be, you may want to extend your sitting time, perhaps up to forty-five minutes or an hour. A longer meditation now and then can be immensely cleansing.

Sitting in a relaxed, yet alert, posture is important. The best position, if you can do it, is to sit cross-legged with a small pillow, such as a Zen *zafu*, under your buttocks. This helps align your spine, and keeps the energy "channel" that runs up and down your spinal column fully open. If you have a physical disability, or very stiff joints, you may find it better to sit in a chair. Again, keep your spine as straight as possible, always taking care not to strain.

Then, once you're sitting, breathe deeply a few times. With your eyes open, take in your environment. Use the breathing to get centered in your body, to allow your energy to gather, so that your attention becomes more at one with the present moment. Let your eyes be soft. Allow yourself to gently receive the visual impressions coming at you. This helps connect you more intimately with your environment.

Then experiment with what George Leonard, an *aikido* master, author, and workshop leader, calls "hard" eyes. Narrow your gaze. Notice how this brings your ego more into play. Notice how "hard" eyes tend to separate you from what you behold. Your look is more piercing. You're more selective, more judgmental in what you choose to see or not see. There's a place for "hard" eyes, especially when you're trying to focus or concentrate on something. Meditation, however, is primarily about letting go of efforting and trying, and instead being fully receptive to what is being felt, seen, heard.

Simply Be Open To What Is

Spend part of your meditation time with your eyes closed, so that you're more attuned to your inner experience. Don't try to stop your thoughts, or fight them. This only creates conflict. Rather, just let them be there, within the space of your awareness, your presence. You're watching them, witnessing them. You're simply open, and in the openness that you are, thoughts, images, and sensations can freely come or go.

Don't get too concerned about what the thought or feeling may be, either. Just be aware that these phenomena are surfacing. In the *vipassana* technique you're taught to not get involved in the content of thoughts, but to simply note that you're thinking, as in, "Oh, thinking again!"

It's easier, too, to witness your thoughts more dispassionately if you start with observing your body's sensations and feelings. When you pay attention to the feedback your body is giving you, you're bringing your awareness down from your forehead, your mind, *into* your body. This is the quickest way to free yourself from distracting thoughts.

When a strong or compelling thought—or sensation, or feeling—does come in, just let it be there. Don't run off with it. Don't let it take you away. Just come back to your breathing, to the feeling of being fully present. Be open to everything. Resist nothing. Allow everything to wash through your awareness, like those birds gliding by. You're not trying to catch them, and you're not following them with your gaze. You're just watching them come and go.

Periodically, open your eyes again. Reconnect with your surroundings. This will help you stay present. There are some who say that the open-eyed meditation, where there's no difference between your inner and outer experience, is the supreme meditation. This is especially so in *dzogchen*, considered by some adepts to be the highest and purest form of Tibetan Buddhist meditation.

I can personally attest to the liberating power of meditating with eyes open. Having your eyes closed can produce illuminating inner experiences, but there still tends to be a sense of a "you" having the experience—following a current of bliss, getting lost in vast spaces, or whatever. When you meditate with open eyes, there's less of that "you" doing or experiencing anything. There's more a feeling of pure openness, limitlessness... *beingness*.

Kundalini and Other Phenomena

It doesn't matter, in the end, whether your eyes are open or shut. Both have value in terms of self-realization. Both teach you important things. Play around with the two modes. Experiment. Make it fun! And remember your goal: to become more and more an unshakable presence, the witness to all that is happening.

Your goal is to be supremely detached, and yet totally present too. Everything happens, unfolds in your awareness. You hold on to none of it. Thoughts, feelings, and sensations arise and disappear again. Sometimes you may experience phenomena such as brilliant lights or colors, sounds, images, tremors, or other manifestations of energy.

You may get a rush of *kundalini*, energy which bursts forth from the base of the spine, the root *chakra*, and ascends toward the crown. Such experiences can be illuminating, shattering, healing, transforming. It's important to just let them be there, to let them pass through you. If you can do that, and stay present with your breath, your body, these dramatic effects will eventually disappear. You'll be left with a deepening sense of clarity, peace, oneness.

In some cases, *kundalini* awakenings can have a negative effect, and leave the meditator feeling agitated and alarmed. It can produce what is known as a "spiritual emergency," a temporary psychosis, where the individual feels panicked, confused, disconnected from reality. If this ever happens to you, seek out professional help. Choose a psychotherapist or skilled teacher who understands meditation and energy phenomena, and who is experienced in addressing these problems.

The more grounded you are in your body, and the more able you are to face and breathe through intense feelings without being overcome by fear, the less of a problem these disturbances will be.

The Attachment to Bliss

Bliss and ecstasy are wonderful by-products of meditation. They are the reward, usually, of many, many hours of sitting and clearing. As you release the blocks and contractions in your body and mind, you'll open more to the energy of spiritual presence itself. This presence is often felt in the cells as a sensation of pure bliss, delight. It's very nourishing and healing. Welcome it and appreciate it when it's there.

Become attached to blissful or ecstatic experiences, however, and you're trapping yourself in an illusion—one that will eventually lead to conflict and unhappiness. The point of meditation is to free yourself from conflict, from all that binds you. When you attach to the feeling of bliss or any other seductive state, you start to get frustrated when the state isn't there. You find yourself getting upset when you can't meditate at your regular time, or when your meditation is disturbed. Sometimes it's a hard truth to admit, but the attachment to bliss or states of any kind is really no different than if you were addicted to a drug, and got upset because you couldn't get your "fix."

When you start to use meditation as an escape from the problems and hard realities of life—rather than as a process for helping you come more fully *into* life—you're headed on a sure path to suffering. It's all too tempting to use meditation to hide out, especially once you've learned how to relax into a tranquil, serene state. Bliss has its joys, but it also has its limitations. It is, after all, only a state—one band-width on the infinite wavelength of life.

This became clear in my own experience. I went through quite a long period where I was very attached to the meditative state. It became relatively easy for me to sit down and feel waves of bliss rolling through my body. The more attached I became to the bliss, the more conflict I experienced in regular life—especially in my marriage and family, and at times when dealing with the world and with business. I remember when my son, Adam, was a baby. I'd sometimes be sitting enjoying my morning meditation, just moving into a state of deep peace and contentment, and suddenly he'd start crying for attention.

Then Barbara, his mother, would call to me from down the hall: "Jim! Adam's diaper needs changing. Please take care of it!" Immediately, I'd contract. "Damn it all!" I'd think to myself, trying to hold on to the bliss I felt. "Why can't she do it? I'm just starting to get comfortable here."

But I'd always get up, grudgingly, and go and take care of Adam's diapers. As much as I resisted it, I knew even then that changing my son's diapers was the real meditation! Indeed, the proof that I was finally making progress in meditation started to become evident when I no longer reacted negatively to such interferences, but got up willingly from my cushion to handle them. I may not have been overjoyed at having my meditation interrupted, but at least I was developing a healthy philosophical acceptance. I was coming more to terms with life's little realities.

After a while, I came to value clarity, openness, and the feeling of being free of all attachments, more than any state of bliss. In this freedom and openness, I discovered, was the peace I'd been seeking all my life. And the beautiful thing about it was that it depended on nothing—not on any thought, belief, or technique. Truly, it did exist on its own.

The Healing Power of Meditation

As it becomes easier and more natural for you to sit in meditation, you'll find that there's a purification that happens with longer sittings, a deep cleansing and renewing in body and mind. You start to get clearer and clearer, and this clarity begins to accompany you more and more throughout the day. You'll also find that when you need guidance on how to deal with a particular problem, longer sittings will be more helpful. In fact, you'll learn to love your daily periods of meditation, both because of the spiritual nourishment you receive, and because of the healing that will take place at all levels of your being.

You'll notice that, just through sitting and being attentive, you can often process and clear the kinds of problems that many people grapple with in psychotherapy for years and years. And the beautiful thing about the meditative approach, why it can be so healing, is that you're not "doing" it. It's not an intellectual or analytical process. You're simply sitting and opening up space for the unresolved material within you, your deeper conflicts and problems, to surface into your awareness—in much the same way as restful sleep can pave the way for dreams that are a source of healing and integration.

It was Albert Einstein who said, "You can't solve a problem at the level of the problem." You have to get some detachment from the problem, in other words. You have to get some perspective in order to see it clearly. Meditation can serve as an invitation, then, for these problems to come up from the deeper regions of consciousness.

In your clear, detached frame of mind, you can acknowledge the existence of the problem. This means you're no longer denying it or repressing it. Instead, you're accepting it, you're fully embracing the realness of it. Then it's a matter of waiting for your higher Self, your inner knowing, to indicate to you, through intuition or insight, what, if anything, you need to do about it at this time. (And, sometimes, the guidance will be to just wait. You'll realize that there's nothing to be done right now).

It's best not to use meditation for guidance in this way until you're able to get into that clear, expanded space fairly easily—until meditation begins to flow naturally for you. If you try to use it for this purpose when your body and mind are still restless or distracted, you're liable to end up with confusing information—which will only make you even more restless!

Focus on finding peace and tranquillity first. Make that your initial goal in meditation, and then later on experiment with using some of your meditative time for problem-solving.

Moving beyond Techniques

Regardless of how long you sit, there will be days when you won't be aware of time at all. Sitting for an hour will feel as though you just sat for ten or fifteen minutes. You'll truly be in that "timeless" place. (And how wonderful it feels to be there!). It helps too, to sit at or near the same time each day. Then your body's biological clock gets used to it. It prepares itself for this period of daily communion with spirit, with your deeper Self.

If you have some experience with meditation, by all means use whatever technique or method you may have learned to help you get still and centered. As your meditation, your inner quiet, deepens, however, you'll probably want to let go of all techniques and methods. Techniques are based upon thought, upon certain ideas or beliefs as to what is effective. So long as you're using a technique— whether a *mantra*, a visualization, counting the breath, or something else—an element of thinking, however subtle, is involved. And wherever there is thinking, or effort, there's the "thinker"—the ego, the personal self, the "me."

The goal in meditation is to get beyond psychological thought, beyond the ego. It's to transcend the active, thinking mind—the personal self, the "me" with all its concerns and desires—and awaken to a deeper spiritual reality. So long as your small "I," your ego, is present in the picture practicing a technique or method, you'll be limited as to how far you can go in your meditation. The deepest and fullest sense of peace and well-being comes in those moments when "you" aren't there.

Meditating with Others

Sometimes people ask me about the value of meditating in groups. The main advantage is that if there's a reasonable degree of unity, of shared purpose and connectedness present in the group, then together you can often experience a deep and powerful meditation. With this in mind, the disadvantage speaks for itself: if the group is restless, if it's without leadership (whether collective or individual), or if the energy is unclear or contracted, it can have a negative, limiting effect on your own meditation.

There's a great benefit to be gained from meditating in the company of someone who is already awake, however. When you're with such a person, there's a transmission that occurs. The clarity and peace emanating from him or her touches you. You get it by osmosis, as it were. Consider yourself blessed if you have a friend, or a spiritual teacher or mentor, who is able to help you awaken to spirit in this way.

Prayer

At this point you may be wondering where prayer fits in with meditation, or the contemplative path. Again, I can only speak of my own experience and understanding. When I was a child, and then as a young man, before I had a really conscious experience of my own divinity—the divinity that's in all of us—I used to communicate with God, or spirit, through prayer. Taking time to pray was always a special and meaningful ritual for me. I didn't know who or what God really was, but I had an intuitive trust in His existence, and that He was there, watching over me.

Once I began to discover true inner silence, however, I felt less and less need for prayer. I had always prayed either to gain peace of mind, or to express my gratitude to God for the blessings in my life. As my meditation deepened, I felt myself more naturally at peace, and my heart overflowed with profound gratitude. In a very real sense, my prayers—even before they were spoken—were already being answered, and so there was no longer any need or desire to pray. Meditation gave me a feeling of fullness and abundance. There was no sense of lack of any kind, so what was the need to pray?

But as life continued to test me in different ways, I found myself developing a new understanding of prayer. I learned that it could be a wonderful way of reconnecting with God, with that sense of universal wisdom and guidance, especially when I was facing a problem I didn't know how to deal with. My favorite prayer for a long time was, simply, "Thy will be done." If I was seeking a certain result, but saw the need for keeping my ego and self-will out of it, I'd pray like this: "Lord, my heart has spoken. You know my wish—and I leave the outcome in your hands." It's a prayer that I still use, on occasion, to this day.

Also, when something particularly special happens—such as one of those miracles that bless us all from time to time—I often find myself spontaneously putting my hands together in thanks, and whispering a prayer of gratitude. Somehow, in doing this, I deepen my capacity to receive the love and goodness that's available to each of us, if we can but open our hearts to it.

Whether you pray or not then, is entirely up to you. There's no "right" way or "wrong" way to do this work of opening to spirit. What I can guarantee you is that the more you commit yourself to taking time each morning for meditation, prayer, reflection, the more you'll benefit from your commitment. As you explore your solitude, your alone time, more deeply, you'll gradually get beyond the worries and concerns of your personal self. You'll open up more fully to the experience of true spiritual freedom.

Returning to Your Natural State of Ease

In this way, meditation becomes an extraordinarily healing adventure. When your mind and body are given a chance to become quiet and still, your physical, mental, and emotional energies are able to reorganize, to re-orchestrate themselves. Like muddied water that begins to clear as soon as it's allowed to settle, so any conflicting energies within you gradually calm down. They naturally and organically distill themselves into a clear, harmonious flow.

Very often, after a ten or twenty minute period of meditation, any pain, stiffness or tension you may have been experiencing—whether in your body or your mind—will magically disappear, and there will be a heightened sense of well-being. After having experienced this enough times, you begin to trust the process. You begin to accept that ease and well-being are your natural state—and that the way back to the truth within you is through letting go of all ideas and images that are not "you."

This, in essence, is the art of meditation. It's releasing all the beliefs, all the mental and emotional programming that's clung to you over the years, so that you can discover what's underneath it all. And what is underneath, you'll sooner or later find (if you persevere, and stay with the process), is a bottomless well of inspiration, strength, and love.

Eventually, if you go far enough in your meditation, you come to the point where your meditative awareness—that sense of infinitude, of being one with the beauty and mystery of life—is not just confined to sitting and being in a quiet and lovely place. More and more it becomes your way of life, your natural state of consciousness, and you bring that quality of attention and sensitivity—with all its potential for healing—to whatever you're doing.

Learning to accept yourself—all those character traits you've judged as negative or unworthy, as well as the positive qualities you may have felt shy about owning—frees you from self-doubt, and brings confidence and peace of mind.

Chapter 10

Accept Yourself

As you've seen in previous chapters, the way to move contracted energy is to breathe into it, and give it space to work itself out.

Another way of describing this is to *accept* what is happening. In accepting something, you're no longer resisting it. Resistance, in one form or another, is the cause of all conflict. The root meaning of the word conflict is "a striking together." A conflict is where two or more forces meet each other head on. The energy given off by their clashing results in the "sparks"—the anger, the upset, the pain, the disturbance—that is experienced as conflict.

At the personal level, you can't be in conflict about a situation unless you're holding on to some belief or viewpoint which is causing you to resist what is. Reality is what it is, whether you like it or not. As you've begun to see, especially in the realm of feelings and emotions, when energy states are accepted as they are, when they are allowed to *be*, it's in their nature to change, to move toward wholeness, or resolution. Such resolution is an expression of the organic unfolding of the life force.

Much of what we in the West have learned from Eastern spiritual traditions such as yoga, Zen, and Taoism, revolves around this notion of acceptance, of being in harmony with what is. This is where the term "going with the flow" comes from. It's to not push the river, to not resist what is happening.

The Taoists call this *wu-wei*, which means non-action, but non-action as the highest form of alertness, of being totally present to what is. This is the wisdom of *wu-wei*. Out of this seemingly passive yet extraordinarily alert quality of attention comes right action—action that is never too much nor too little, but rather always appropriate to the situation at hand.

An image from the East that is often used is that of bamboo. A bamboo stalk is firmly rooted, anchored in the ground, so that even in the strongest wind it won't blow over or break. It is supple and flexible. It is able to bend with the wind. This is the secret of its stability and its longevity. No matter which direction the wind blows, the bamboo can bend with it and then, when the force of the wind is spent, it springs back to its normal, upright position.

The bamboo image is a helpful one to remember when you're practicing grounding and centering yourself. It is to see and feel your feet as the roots of the bamboo, firmly planted on the earth. The rest of your body—your steady but relaxed legs, your unlocked knees, your balanced pelvis, your soft belly, your loose shoulders, your alert gaze—is like the stalk of the bamboo, pliable, firm, yielding, and strong.

Creating Out of Wholeness Versus Conflict

When Westerners first encounter these concepts of non-resistance, harmony, and flow, they often struggle against them—in a typically Western way! People in the West, especially in highly technological cultures like the U.S., are used to controlling and manipulating their environment, and their circumstances. They are accustomed to clashing egos and interpersonal conflict, and often derive tremendous energy from it. The emphasis on individual personality, on ego, is much stronger in the West than in the East, where people tend to live more in harmony with the natural, organic rhythms and movements of life. It's no surprise that Westerners seeking inner peace frequently end up looking to the East.

To create from this kind of tension or conflict is one way of producing creative works, but it doesn't necessarily bring about a heightened state of well-being in the person doing it. Think of the many artists, composers, and writers the West has produced who, though they brought forth great works of art, suffered much unhappiness within themselves, and often ended their lives in despair.

There's a different way to create, to compose, write or paint, and that is to do it out of wholeness. Many Western artists are in touch with the beauty and wholeness of life, and this comes through in their work, yet they fail, so often, to find that balance in their own lives. In Zen it is said that if you want to paint a beautiful picture, first be a beautiful person, and then paint naturally. Discover wholeness, or unity, within yourself, and out of that sense of integration within, create something meaningful and beautiful with your life.

Spiritual paths like Zen have a lot to teach us about healing. Zen is really concerned with the art of living a happy, peaceful, and productive life. It's not just to go through your life passively, accepting whatever comes your way—as many Westerners may think when they contemplate the image of an Oriental man or woman quietly sweeping the path, trimming a bonsai, or arranging flowers in a lovely display. Rather, Zen is about awakening to your deeper nature, your Buddha-nature—the eternal wisdom of life which expresses through you, and which governs the unfolding of all creation—and then learning to live your life out of that understanding.

You may prefer to attribute this wisdom to God, Grace, or whatever you call the higher power that governs the universe. In the grand scheme of things it doesn't matter much what name you use. All words, regardless of how exalted or appealing they may be, are only concepts anyway. When you strip away the concepts, the beliefs and names, what you're left with is the timeless rhythm of life and creation, of night dissolving into day, of the seasons following one another, of rainy days and dry, of birth, growth, death, and rebirth.

To realize you are one with that rhythm, to learn how to dance with it, to harness its creative power so that you can do something meaningful with your life, something that contributes to the well-being of others, is what Zen teaches. It is the deeper promise of our own Judeo-Christian tradition too, if we would but probe beneath the surface religious conditioning most of us have received. Jesus' whole message was about living in the present, listening to an inner voice and, rather than hiding one's light, letting it shine forth in the form of love and good works.

The True Meaning of Surrender

Acceptance, then, isn't simply giving up or passively surrendering to someone or something, but rather it's a way of really *being* with the moment at hand. It's learning to develop rapport, the ability to flow with the situation so that you learn from it. Then you're open to the creative potential that is always present, just as the master potter allows the feel of the spinning clay in his hands to guide his touch, and tell him what shape it wants to take.

Some have called this process *co-creation*. You're working directly with the forces before you. You might like to think of it as co-creating with God, or with the Tao. Again, the way into co-creation is through acceptance, through not struggling against what is. It's to welcome the totality of your experience, to embrace it. You can't embrace anything so long as you are still resisting it, or fighting it.

Conflict, if it persists, leads to suffering. If it continues unabated, it can hurt you, make you ill. Prolonged conflict tears you up inside, and wrenches people apart. Long-term emotional stress takes a toll on the body. When two people in a relationship are unable to meet in harmony, the relationship degenerates.

Conflict can serve a purpose, however. It can act as a signal, a pointer back towards wholeness, if you'll but heed the message. It shows you where the healing is needed in your life. The challenge is to learn to acknowledge the fact of conflict early on, and then to do something about it, to look for the resolution. This is how you learn from conflict.

In acknowledging the conflict, you're coming out of denial around it. You are accepting the reality of it. In acceptance, there's an integration of energy. When you stop fragmenting your energy through denial and non-acceptance, you see what's in front of you more clearly. By surrendering, or giving up your judgments, opinions, and expectations, you get more insight into what is *actually* going on—into the nature of the conflict. You get information about it. This clear seeing then leads to right action.

It's similar to when you're dealing with a young child who is proving difficult, perhaps even on the verge of a tantrum. If you try to make the child be quiet, force him or her to be still, you'll almost assuredly meet with resistance. There will be a clash of wills. But if you accept that acting out emotionally is what the child needs to do right now, and give space for that young, vital energy to expend itself—while at the same time providing safe boundaries for it—the child will eventually calm down. The tide of explosive, volatile energy will ebb, and then you'll be able to talk with the child in a way that will increase the chances of both of you being heard.

Practice letting go of your resistance to the events and circumstances in your life, and you'll be surprised at how much smoother and more effortlessly your days will proceed.

Stop Fighting Yourself

Learning to dance with energy in this way, to not resist circumstances or conditions, but rather to work with them in order to accomplish your goals and objectives, teaches you about self-acceptance. To accept yourself means you're no longer fighting yourself, you're no longer doubting yourself. You're no longer at war within yourself.

Coming to genuine self-acceptance is the first enlightenment, the one that paves the way for the realization and embodiment of your true spiritual nature. Once you accept yourself, then you are free to be all of who you are. So long as you continue to fight yourself, however, you are dividing and wasting your energy, and you won't find the focus, the sense of a deeper purpose in life, you've been seeking.

Self-acceptance begins with self-observation. It's to pay attention to how you feel, and especially, what you *think* about how you feel—the ways in which you may judge yourself, compare yourself, or put yourself down. When you label yourself as bad, inferior or "less than," or when you tell yourself something like, "I shouldn't feel like this," or "I shouldn't be like this," or "I don't like the way I look," it indicates that you're rejecting something about yourself.

Rejection is a form of resisting what is so. It is looking at a fact, something that exists, and saying, "No, I don't want to believe this, I don't want to look at this, I don't want to accept this." It's a denial of reality, and so long as it goes on it will cause conflict. Denial or resistance of this kind gives rise to chronic self-doubt and uncertainty. It's very disempowering. It erodes your confidence and leaves you frustrated, unfulfilled, resentful.

To heal yourself, you must start accepting reality as it is. Only when you accept the existence of something—whether a feeling, a thought, a circumstance, or a situation—can you then blend its energy into your own. To unify energy in this way is empowering. You become stronger. You're no longer dissipating energy in resistance and conflict.

You must learn to accept it all then—all that you feel, all that you think, all that you are. "Welcome your experience," as Jean Klein says. Embrace it. If you're critical or judgmental, acknowledge the fact, accept it and you will soon find yourself being less judgmental. This happened to me many years ago. A close friend pointed out to me, during a conversation, that I tended to be very judgmental toward other people. For some reason—perhaps just because I was ready—I was able to hear it. In fact, I responded by exclaiming, "God, you're right! I am judgmental, aren't I?"

It was a revelation to me. Thereafter, I became acutely aware every time I judged someone in that old, critical way of mine. More importantly, I began to accept that I had this habit—without judging myself for it! I saw the connection between judging others and being hard on myself. As I started to be easier on myself, so I was easier on others.

To use good judgment in terms of making wise choices and decisions is healthy. But to be judgmental in the sense of putting yourself and others down only hardens you. It cuts you off from your feelings, your natural sensitivity. It closes down your heart, and gets in the way of your experiencing real closeness with people. If you're a judgmental type of person, start looking at the emotional wounds, the pain from your past, that has caused you to armor yourself in this way. Stop judging yourself and just feel your pain. Love yourself. Let the judgments go.

Getting free of judgment is an essential step to freedom.

The Art of Defusing Conflict

If you don't like something about yourself, acknowledge how you feel. Say to yourself, "I realize I really don't like this about myself." Accept the fact that you don't like it. Learn to live with the not-liking. Let it be there. Let it be there with whatever feelings may be accompanying it. Stop resisting what is so, and how you feel about what is so, and a day will come when it won't be such an issue.

When you stop resisting what you're experiencing and begin instead to accept it, to allow the thought or feeling to just be there, it takes the emotional charge off it. It defuses it, in the same way that an *aikido* master, when being attacked, literally "accepts" the attacker's energy, allows the person to come into his space.

The *aikidoist* dances with the attacker, in effect, utilizing the assailant's energy to defeat him. When the dance is over the aggressor is lying helpless on the ground, while the master is still standing. It's a paradox at first glance, but the master remains fully in control of the situation by giving up control, by allowing a deeper law, or principle of harmony, to operate instead.

The law is that energy follows the path of least resistance. What this means is that the stronger the resistance you give to a force, the more you block the flow, or the energy, of that force. This creates a clash of energies: the energy behind your resistance, and the energy of the force coming at you. Because of the clash, you have a conflict. If you've ever been locked in an argument with a strong-willed person, you'll know what I mean!

The *aikido* expert understands this principle, and spends his life mastering it. His whole art is based upon it, which is why it's so powerful. When he meets an opposing force, he doesn't try to stop it or overwhelm it. To do so would involve an unnecessary expenditure of energy on his part—and, if the attacker were stronger, might even result in harm to himself.

So what the master does is put up no resistance at all. He simply offers a little bit of direction for the energy coming at him. He grasps the person's wrist, steps to one side, gives a quick and subtle flick and—presto!—the assailant finds himself being driven straight into the ground. The violent momentum behind the attack is channelled exactly where the master wants it, following the path of least resistance. This is a beautiful example of *wu-wei*, or not-doing, in action.

Owning Your Feelings and Desires

One of the main forms of resistance and conflict you'll experience is around feelings and desires. You may find yourself desiring solitude, for example, and yet someone close to you is seeking your company, and perhaps trying to make you feel guilty for wanting to be alone. Or you may desire to be successful in some way—whether financially, or in terms of career advancement, or a project you're working on—and others are telling you it's not possible, or you won't be able to do it and maintain your integrity.

Or your desires may revolve around other activities or pursuits, to do with friendship, sex, spirituality, living a certain lifestyle, satisfying a curiosity, or expressing yourself in some way that is important or meaningful for you. It doesn't really matter what the desire is. Desires only become a problem when you experience conflict around them, when words like "should," "should not," "can't" or "forbidden" enter your reality, and cause you to reject or struggle with what you're feeling.

To resolve these kinds of conflicts, you must first see that the resistance to what you're feeling, all the beliefs and judgments around it, come from within you. Others may reinforce what you're thinking and feeling through their opinions and attitudes, but you can't hold them responsible for what's going on inside you. Remember, you're the source of your own inner experience. You're the one in charge of your life. You're the one who decides, ultimately, what is good for you. No one else can do that for you.

When you were a child, others—your parents, primarily—did have power over you. Their beliefs and attitudes helped shape your world-view, as well as your self-image. You received most of your values from your parents. The judgments you've acquired about what's acceptable and what's not, came largely from those who raised you.

Like most people, you've probably allowed those values and the beliefs behind them to run your life ever since. But now, here you are, on this journey of transformation. You may be at a point in your life where you've been through some significant changes, or have suffered a major loss, or are experiencing doubts about what you want to do with yourself in the future. In psychological language, you may be going through an identity crisis.

This is the time when your world-view, and the beliefs behind it, is most susceptible to change. You are beginning to see their limitation, that they aren't really serving you. They have outlived their usefulness, their workability. They limit your creativity. They don't allow for the full expression of who you are. They are old patterns, and your insistence on clinging to them is preventing anything new and authentic from emerging.

Before you can let anything go, however, you must be aware that you're holding onto it. You must own it, or accept it. And this applies equally to any desires you may have. Before you can get free of them, or get free of the conflict around them, you must allow yourself to have them. Otherwise you'll continue to live in denial. You'll fail to see what is really going on—and what needs to change—in your life.

Self-acceptance begins with owning your feelings and desires. It's taking responsibility for what you're experiencing. Others may try to impose their will, their beliefs and judgments on you, but you must understand that what you're experiencing is *your* experience. Listen to the feedback you get from others, by all means, but then look inside and do a reality check. Ask yourself, "What's really true for me?"

Trust the guidance that follows. You may be unclear, you may even be mistaken at times, but the more you practice trusting yourself, the stronger your trust will become.

Seeing Your Own Beauty

When you blame others for your discontent or unhappiness, you disempower yourself. This tendency to put it all on the shoulders of another as a way of avoiding yourself is known in psychology as "projection." It's something most of us do unconsciously. It is far easier to point the finger at another's faults, at someone else's personality flaws, than to live with the discomfort of our own. Yet healing is about becoming more conscious. Before you can truly accept yourself, you have to own your projections. You have to bring everything back home.

A useful exercise for learning self-acceptance is to take some time each day to look into a mirror and just be with yourself, with everything you see, and with the feelings that come up. For many people, this is a very difficult exercise. They can look into a mirror to shave, brush their hair, apply their make-up, or attend to their appearance in some other way, but this is a more superficial looking. The focus here is on image, on the outer, and not on the inner reality.

If this exercise proves difficult for you, if it brings up too much emotional discomfort or self-judgment, it shows that you still have some work to do on self-acceptance. In this case, try the exercise for only a few minutes at a time. Do it for as long as you can stand it, and come back to the mirror at another time.

You are learning to be vulnerable with yourself, open to any painful judgments and feelings you may have previously been repressing. It takes strength and courage to be open in this way. Only a person who really accepts and trusts him or herself can afford to be vulnerable. This is why the *Course In Miracles*, a text which focuses on guiding readers back to the love within them, instructs, "In my defenselessness my safety lies." Understand the meaning behind that statement, and you'll have one of the main keys to inner peace.

Don't be concerned about being narcissistic, either. Narcissus was a mythological character who fell in love with his own reflection. People who are very self-absorbed are enamored of their own reflection. They are forever checking their appearance in the mirror, and are constantly obsessed with the image they present to the world. You're learning to get beyond image and reflection so that you can discover something deeper within you, something authentic—your real Self.

During your "mirror meditation" make sure you remember to breathe whenever any tension or uneasiness arises. Look into your eyes. Really see yourself. Smile at yourself. Honor your wrinkles, your facial lines. You've earned them! Practice frowning. Laugh.

Scowl. Screw your face up. Notice what kinds of feelings or emotions these expressions may evoke within you.

Consider how you feel about yourself, how you rate yourself on the self-esteem scale. Think of certain people you may like or dislike, or recall incidents from the past that may be emotionally-charged for you, and see what effect that has. Again, the idea is to just be present with yourself, to see if you can stay with yourself throughout this process, and not run away.

Self-acceptance means not abandoning yourself, even when the feelings get uncomfortable or intense. Much of the loneliness we feel comes about not because others have deserted us, as we would like to think, but because we have abandoned ourselves. To accept yourself is to really be there for yourself. It's learning to be your own best friend.

Notice the judgments you may have about yourself as you practice this mirror meditation. Let the judgments be there. Say to yourself, "Yes, I have these judgments, and there's nothing wrong with having them. Everybody has judgments. The more I acknowledge and accept them, the less they control me, and the freer I am."

Think about the various desires you have, the ones that excite you or please you, and those that make you feel guilty or confused. Again, say to yourself, "I have these desires, and there's nothing wrong with them. Every human being has had these desires at one time or another. I have the power to choose whether to act on them or not."

This is also a time when you can think about the mistakes you may have made in your life, the poor decisions, the "wrong" choices. To accept yourself is to forgive yourself. It is to be grateful for the lessons you are learning, the lessons yet to come. Perhaps you're feeling stuck. There may be no movement, nothing new or productive happening in your life. Can you look at yourself in the mirror and acknowledge the fact that you feel stuck? That perhaps you don't know what to do at this time, that you may not even know what you want to do? Accepting where you are takes the pressure off yourself. Then you can breathe more easily and see more clearly.

Lastly, can you accept conflict and uncertainty itself? This is what really counts. It's being able to look at yourself in the mirror and simply be with your discomfort. It's a matter of softening your belly, of opening your heart, of being gentle with yourself.

It's to say to yourself, as you view your reflection in the mirror, "You're okay, you know. I love you, and I'm learning to feel good about who you are. I'm learning to accept you as you are."

Self-Acceptance Sets You Free

The more you can just be with yourself in this way, the less you will struggle in life. Self-acceptance opens the door to a deeper, richer, and more satisfying experience of living. It's the great peacemaker, the true emotional healer. If you practice the mirror exercise regularly, there will come a day when you'll be able to look at yourself without any negative reaction at all. You'll smile, give a nod, and simply appreciate both the beauty and the ordinariness of your own being.

The beauty will show through not because you've finally eliminated or gotten rid of all your flaws and imperfections, but because you've *accepted* these things about yourself. You'll have integrated them into the totality of your being—"All of this is who I am, and it's all okay."

It's a marvelous freedom to no longer be at war with yourself. It allows you to have more compassion for others. You'll be able to see their beauty more readily, even when they can't see it themselves. Your own self-acceptance will inspire them. They will sense you are at ease with yourself, and this will help them relax. Through self-acceptance, you heal both yourself and your relationships.

To truly accept yourself is, in the end, to transcend yourself. It's to rise above the limitations of egocentric thinking, of endlessly thinking about "I," "me," and "mine." You come to the place where you don't think about yourself as much any more. You cease being obsessed with your own psychological and emotional process—and especially your "spiritual" progress! Truly, there is nowhere to get to, and there is no special way to be. You're just being yourself, living your life, doing what you love.

It may help you to understand what it means to live without "self" concern by considering what happens when you watch a movie you're enjoying. Because the movie interests you, you're totally absorbed in it. You're not sitting back distant from it, judging it, feeling restless, wondering if it's going to get better and whether you should stick it out, or leave. There's no "you" there. You're completely immersed in the drama playing itself out on the screen. Yet you're still yourself, and if you were to pause and sit back for a moment to notice how you felt, you'd be aware of a wholly nourishing, satisfying experience. An experience of wholeness, of being complete.

In Zen it is said, "When you look into a mirror and you see no one there, then you've found enlightenment." What is meant by this is not that there's no reflection looking back at you. There's your face, obviously. But there's no ego in the way, no "me" worrying about how attractive or unattractive it looks, or how rapidly it seems to be aging, or how it's going to pay the bills next month. There's just this person, beaming love and light—its Buddha-nature—back at you.

It's wonderful to experience these moments of freedom, to come to the place where you can look into an "empty" mirror and appreciate just how beautifully simple it all really is. And if someone were to ask you how you came to this peace and confidence you've begun to enjoy, you may find yourself saying with a grin, "It's been a long struggle, but I've finally begun to accept myself for who I am."

Addictions are a form of disempowerment. They support the illusion that the happiness you seek depends on something outside yourself. As you free yourself from your addictions you rediscover the power and strength within you.

Chapter 11

Free Yourself from Addictions

Learning to accept yourself inevitably involves looking at your addictions, the self-defeating habits and behaviors you may be caught in that not only keep you from fulfilling your true creative potential, but may also—if the addiction is severe enough—be causing a real problem in your life.

Cigarette smoking, alcoholism, drug abuse, sexual promiscuity, over-eating, and over-spending are among the most common addictions any of us can fall prey to, but they are not the complete list by any means. You can also, for example, become addicted to pleasing other people, to trying to take care of their feelings at the expense of your own, giving rise to the behavior known as "co-dependency."

You can become addicted to certain beliefs and ideas, to obsessive thinking, so that you end up playing the same mental refrain over and over again, never allowing room for anything new or original to come into your mind. As I pointed out in the chapter on meditation, you can even become addicted to meditation, to the peace and tranquillity you find when you detach yourself from all your worldly responsibilities.

Because of the heightened social awareness of the problem of addiction, the term "recovery" is now part of everyday usage. To be in recovery is to be working toward getting free of addictions. It's to move toward sobriety, to a healthier, saner, more balanced way of living. For many of us, the work done around recovering from addictive habits and behaviors is the most important healing work we undertake. Often it's only our addictions that keep us from experiencing the deeper feeling of well-being we seek.

The word "addiction" means to give over, to surrender yourself to something. It implies being taken over or controlled by a habit or practice of some kind. The forms of addiction are legion. When you're addicted to something, whether it's a physical habit like alcohol or over-eating, or a behavioral one like being emotionally over-reactive in your relationships, or too mental, too analytical in your approach to life, that addiction has you in its grip.

To the extent that you're controlled by an addiction, you can't access your full intuitive and creative resources. Your attention gets fixated on the object of your addiction—the "fix"—and it becomes a distraction. You rely on the addiction to feel a sense of ease within, but it's an artificial state. You can't get down to your true depths. While you may feel relaxed and peaceful for a while—or stimulated, if that's what the addiction does for you—afterward you have to deal with the inevitable side-effects of the substance or habit. This usually means a hangover, upset digestion, depleted energy, an inability to think clearly and to focus your attention, and—very often—feelings of low self-esteem.

But if addictions didn't do something for us, we wouldn't touch them. The physical ones like alcohol, drugs, and food fill up the empty spaces within, they smooth out the rough edges, they take the tension out of life. They give a temporary sense of physical well-being, and with it, a feeling of psychological and emotional ease too.

Emotional addictions do the same thing, in a different way. Sometimes the only way a person can get rid of their emotional tension, the uncomfortable feelings that are so difficult to be with, is to express them reactively through explosive anger or rage. Other people, more repressed in nature, will deal with those same uncomfortable feelings by simply refusing to feel them. Instead, they'll rationalize them away. They'll get lost in a maze of thinking, analysis, and theory—the mind's addiction—as a way of avoiding having to feel what they're actually experiencing in their bodies.

Some people, on the other hand, may not be able to stand silence, the absence of noise or activity. They'll need to talk, or turn on the radio, or do something in order to eliminate the anxiety they feel when things start to get too quiet and still. Or they'll spend hours on the telephone, endlessly discussing their problems with their friends—and usually just going round and round in circles, without actually resolving anything.

Such people are addicted to being busy. They only know themselves, only feel secure within themselves, when there's movement, activity, something happening. Stillness, instead of being an invitation to open up to their feelings and their inner experience, will be perceived as threatening, and even frightening.

We give ourselves over to addictions precisely because of the sense of security and well-being we get from them. Even when we know that the feeling of well-being is temporary, and that the addiction itself may be physically harmful, we persist in going for the short-term benefit. For addictions do fulfill a certain kind of promise. They work. They can be relied on, most of the time, to give us the kind of satisfaction—brief though it may be—that we've come to expect from them.

An Illusory Well-Being

In terms of mental and emotional health, addictions are disempowering because of the way in which they keep you locked into limited and ultimately unfulfilling patterns of behavior. Whenever you depend upon an agent of any kind for your well-being—and this includes beliefs, dogmas, repetitive emotional patterns or habitual ways of thinking, as well as the many physical stimulants—the well-being you experience is never truly yours.

Instead, there's a dependency, which is the nature of addiction. The emotional trap of dependency is that it's a love/hate relationship, and therefore has the potential for producing considerable inner conflict. When you depend on something or someone outside yourself for your well-being, you love it when that thing or person comes through for you. But when it doesn't, you'll notice that you get angry, resentful, anxious. You often end up hating that on which you've come to depend. We've all experienced this addiction to things or people outside ourselves. The fact is that real freedom is not possible as long as there is dependency.

From a spiritual perspective, addictions are disempowering because they reinforce the sense or feeling that you're not enough within yourself, and that to be happy you need something else. You need to fill yourself up with something in order to feel at ease within.

The paradox is that we cling to our addictions because we don't know ourselves spiritually. We don't feel that deep sense of inner well-being which, when we're in touch with it, nourishes and sustains us in a way that no external stimulant ever can. It's no accident, perhaps, that one of the most popular and time-tested approaches to dealing with addiction and the suffering it produces, is the Twelve Step program.

The Twelve Steps

The success of the Twelve Steps, which came out of the Alcoholics Anonymous movement, lies in its recognition of the fact that addictions are symbolic of a spiritual hunger or emptiness. This is why any attempt to free yourself of addictions through willpower are usually self-defeating.

If you're strong-willed enough, you may be successful in eliminating certain addictions, but the chances are that you're still addicted to the sense of "me" and "mine." Strong-willed people are often dominated by their egos. It's the ego, the attachment to our psychological and emotional identity—to the belief that "I control my life"—that causes us to feel separate and apart from spirit, the underlying unity and wholeness of life.

This feeling of separateness, of having to constantly compete and struggle with every other human being for a tenuous security, is the fundamental spiritual dilemma facing us all. It's the conflict that most needs healing. When this healing begins to happen, everything else starts to fall into place. You notice yourself beginning to live your life, finally, as a more integrated human being. You feel connected to something bigger than yourself, and are therefore less afraid of life, less afraid of others. You feel empowered by this larger energy. It helps you get clearer about what you want to do with your life, and you're more capable of actually doing it.

I have a friend whose spiritual path is the Twelve Step program. I have only to look at her to see how well the Twelve Steps can work. She is freer of the suffering that used to plague her. She is more emotionally stable. Her life is more in balance. I see that she blames others less, and is finding a new strength within herself as she takes more responsibility for her own situation. She is less interested in the kind of immediate but short-term gratification that her addictions used to offer, and more committed to doing the work necessary to find a more constant well-being.

She is a happier person, and much more present in body, mind, and soul than when I first knew her. She is less distracted, less self-obsessed—the mark of the willful, addicted person—and much more surrendered to a deeper wisdom, to what the Twelve Steps call "a Power greater than ourselves."

It's a paradox, but in learning to surrender her will to this Higher Power, she has found herself more empowered at a personal level. She has begun to embody the spirit of that great liberating prayer, "Not my will, O Lord, but Thine." In her own way she is going through a genuine spiritual awakening, and it's gradually transforming her life.

You may find that your own spiritual practice is inspired by a tradition other than the Twelve Steps. Yet, if you really look at it, you'll probably notice there's not a lot of difference between the route you may take and that preferred by my friend, and so many others who have sought to heal themselves through the Twelve Steps.

All of us committed to the healing journey are heading toward the same place. We're learning to be more ordinary, to be simpler, to be humbler. We're learning to be more grateful as we wake up each morning, and realize that God—the wisdom and power behind existence—has given us yet another chance at life, at becoming a better and more whole human being.

The Twelve Steps work because they are founded on truth. They recognize that spiritual freedom only comes as you get free of the limitations of your personal self—the endless cycle of self-centered thinking—and open up to something bigger than you. But to have a program like the Twelve Steps, or any spiritual practice, actually make a difference in your life, you have to commit to it and follow it. You have to work at it.

Having a Personal Program

Having a program to follow is of the utmost importance. I see this time and time again in my practice. It doesn't matter what the issue or the goal is, either. It's the people who exercise regularly, who are conscious of what they eat, and who pay attention to the relationship between mental attitude and stress, who have the fewest problems with their bodies. They not only have fewer problems, they actually begin to feel stronger and healthier in every way. It often surprises them because they didn't know they could feel so well. Their energy felt so low, or they were so out of shape for so many years, they had begun to think it was normal.

A personal program of spiritual development brings similar results. Some days will be easier than others. Sometimes it will be very difficult to stay centered, to remember your connection with your Higher Power, or whatever you call that energy which is at the source of life. At such times phrases like "Thy will, not mine," "Let go and let God," or "One day at a time," can often help. These are simple, proven affirmations, ones which you've probably heard many times, and yet when said with feeling, with meaning, they can be enormously beneficial.

After all, sobering up, learning to live a more sane and balanced life, can be a very painful experience. Whether you're freeing yourself from addiction to alcohol or drugs, or over-eating, or emotional excess, or financial irresponsibility, or the bliss of escaping into altered states of consciousness, there's a detoxification process you'll have to go through. The detoxification may involve the elimination of actual poisons and impurities from your body if the addiction is to a physical substance (in which case nutritional support can be of great value). Or it may be the equally painful letting go of your illusions and fantasies as you wake up, finally, to all that you've been missing in life.

Sobriety, or being an ordinary human being living an ordinary, useful life, can at first seem quite boring and unfulfilling. You may find yourself missing the highs that you so loved—the excitement, the juice, the intensity, and the adrenaline that once made living seem so special.

My own addiction for many years was the bliss of meditation and related transcendent experiences. Having grown up in a home where there was frequently an undercurrent of conflict and tension, I became addicted to peace and quiet—so much so that I made a practice of avoiding any situation that might be emotionally upsetting.

This avoidance pattern probably caused me to miss, over the years, a lot of potentially creative opportunities. I just didn't want to deal with anything that might involve conflict. In the end, though, I had to face the fact that I was missing out on real growth and learning. There was a lot I wanted to do with my life. I finally saw that I couldn't fulfill my heart's desires as long as I continued to shy away from situations that threatened to push me out of my comfort zone. Letting go of that addiction was difficult—and it didn't happen overnight.

You may start questioning, as I did, the meaning of your life. You may wonder what there is to look forward to now that you've begun to see the limitations of escaping, of getting high, of acting out your old addictive patterns. These kinds of issues will come up as you begin to acknowledge to yourself that it's time to do something different with your life.

The Addiction to Transcendence

One of the most seductive addictions for spiritual seekers is the addiction to transcendence—to rising above pain and suffering. Indeed, all forms of addiction are, in a way, a desire to transcend unwanted experience.

My own addiction to transcendence was brought home to me many years ago, in a vivid and revealing dream I had. In the dream, I was sunbathing, in the nude, on a small island in the river that runs parallel to the road leading into California's Yosemite valley. The river was bounded on both sides by a forest. I was leaning back on a secluded patch of sand, supported by two large, smooth boulders. Then, strangely, the boulders turned into flesh, into the thighs of my mother, and I realized I was experiencing the moment of my birth. I was issuing forth from my mother's womb, about to begin my life in the world.

I was aware of a lot of blood, sweat, and pain as I struggled for my first breath and looked around. All I could see was a mass of suffering of humanity, mirroring my own shock at being so rudely ejected into the world—a world I suddenly wasn't at all sure I wanted to join. People were crying and screaming. They were fighting with each other, desperate in their need to find a place where they belonged, where they could be themselves, where they could find peace. They were making a horrible clamor and were locked in a conflict that showed no signs of ceasing. The more I looked, the worse the noise and distress became. That was enough for me. I staggered to my feet, through the mess of blood and afterbirth.

"Where are you going?" I heard my mother call softly.

"I can't stand all this pain and confusion!" I cried. "I've got to get away!"

"No!" she said, grabbing my arm and pulling me back. "That's why I brought you here. To help clean it up."

I stopped, looked up at the ancient cliffs towering above the side of the Yosemite valley. Something caught my eye. There, high up on a precipice above the pandemonium around me, was the figure of a Zen monk, sitting quietly in serene meditation.

"*That's* where I want to be. Up there!"

I pointed to the monk. My mother relaxed her grip. I started to move toward the base of the cliff. Then, as if by magic, the din around me stopped for a moment. The monk seemed to turn my way, and though he was too far off for me to be sure, I swore he smiled. His voice echoed clearly inside my head: "There's only room for one of us up here, boy."

I sat down, buried my head in my hands. An enormous sadness overtook me. I felt hopeless, helpless. Then I felt my mother's loving arms encircle me, and I awoke from the dream.

That dream stayed with me for many years. It was like a compass, pointing me back to the truth I was still reluctant to hear. I still wanted to believe that I, too, could be up there, far removed from the tumult and suffering of my fellow man. Yet it wasn't to be. The more attached I became to the transcendent peace I found during my periods of meditation, the more the world—and my own suffering in relationship to it—called me back.

The monk was right. A safe mountain refuge was not to be my destiny in this lifetime. And my mother was right. I was here to help clean things up. To help with the healing. My sense is that we're all here for that purpose. None of us can do it alone. We created the mess we find ourselves in. It's up to us to make things right.

The Promise of Sobriety

What you'll discover, as you go further on your healing journey is that being ordinary, living in the everyday world, is not so bad after all. At first, yes, it can be quite disillusioning. It will help if you remember that enlightenment, or spiritual awakening, is really about getting *free* of your illusions, and learning to live in reality.

It's a journey of letting go of those emotionally-charged memories of the past, your fantasies, worries, and concerns about the future, and living more wholeheartedly in the present. As you begin to get in sync with reality, with the way things actually are, your whole perspective on life will begin to shift.

Reality, you'll discover, doesn't have to be ongoing emotional pain and suffering. It doesn't require that you remain in dysfunctional relationships. It doesn't mean that you have to remain the victim of unhealthy addictions and intolerable circumstances. Instead, you begin to realize how much freedom you have to *create* a different reality, once you've aligned yourself with a deeper spiritual purpose.

As you clean up your diet, begin to exercise regularly, meditate each day, and work on healing your relationships, your choices expand and reality starts to take on a different feel. You begin to get a sense of inner serenity, of what it means to be a happy, fulfilled person. You begin to taste what it's like to go through the whole day with an underlying sense of peace and calm, so that the inevitable ups and downs of circumstances don't upset you in the way they did previously.

The more you touch this energy of clarity and harmony, the more you'll want to seek it out. When spiritual well-being becomes your goal, your focus in life, your addictions—the habits and behaviors which were once so self-defeating—naturally begin to fall away.

This is the promise of sobriety, of freeing yourself from addictions. As you discover what it is to be more ordinary, to live a normal, wholesome life, you'll find that you won't want to trade it for all the "highs" in the world. If you're like most people who have worked through the pain of addictions, you'll remember all too well the price you paid for those highs, and for all that erratic, self-destructive behavior.

Besides, you'll undoubtedly find that walking in the world with true balance, with a clear head and a steady heart—and experiencing this on an increasingly consistent basis—is the best feeling there is.

To be assertive, directed, and goal-oriented are the masculine qualities, to be patient, receptive, and nurturing, the feminine. To have both the masculine and the feminine integrated within yourself is to be a whole person.

Chapter 12
Integrate the Masculine and Feminine

As you free yourself from your addictions and awaken to your own spiritual energy, you find yourself becoming more self-contained. You learn to enjoy your own solitude more. It's during your alone times that you'll most likely feel the connection to spirit, your true nature, most deeply. Because of this increasing feeling of autonomy, of being at one with a larger sense of beingness, rather than depending on individual objects or people for your happiness, you may find that you don't need others in quite the same way as you once did.

You do not need them to fill your emotional needs to the same degree, for example, because spirit, the energy within you, takes care of that for you. The connection you're developing with your spiritual self becomes so nourishing that it tends to fill up any "empty" spaces within you. It heals your psychological conflicts. It cleanses your emotional wounds. It will cure many of your physical problems. It will bring an increasingly rich measure of love and joy to your heart.

And yet you'll still have a natural desire for companionship, for friendship and, yes, for intimacy with a special "other," for a partner, a spouse, a lover. Very few of us are cut out to be monks or nuns, or want to spend our entire lives meditating in quiet solitude, far removed from the mass of humanity. True, we want inner peace and a harmonious life, yet we also want to enjoy our embodied existence. We want to taste of all that this beautiful world has to offer us.

The more you feel the love of spirit within you, the more likely you are to want to create relationships where you can share your inner richness with others. You may seek out a spiritual community, for example—if not formally, then certainly in the form of friendships with people who are on the same wave-length as you, who feel the same deep affection for life, the same reverence for the mystery and the beauty of Being, as you do.

In your love relationships, you'll find that the most satisfying communion of all is when you and your lover meet in true spiritual intimacy. In the same way, the most fulfilling sex is the sex that happens when you and your lover are joined in conscious spiritual union. When two lovers are attuned to each other in every cell of their Being, so that there is just the one rhythm, the one current of energy flowing through them, then the chemistry that happens is extraordinary. Then sex is truly a celebration, a consummation, of the love that you feel for each other.

This kind of conscious merging represents what is possible in a man-woman love relationship. You touch these spiritual heights and depths with your lover—or in a conversation with a friend, or during a time of genuine family peace and unity—in very special moments. You cannot control them or make them happen. They only occur when the "controller"—the ego—is out of the way. As a consequence, and because most of us are still dealing with our ego at some level, the dance that goes on in our relationships tends to be much more mundane—and often, ridden with conflict!

In this chapter, and the next, I want to explore the subject of relationship and how, along with meditation and the work you do in the world, it's the most challenging yet potentially productive arena available to you for furthering your growth and healing. To begin, I want to suggest that many—and perhaps most—of the problems encountered in our interpersonal relationships are but a reflection of the unhealed aspects of the relationship we have with ourselves. The outer is a reflection of the inner.

As you've seen in the chapter on self-acceptance, learning to acknowledge and accept the things you don't like about yourself, the traits and habits you've judged as "bad" or "wrong" in some way, is one of the most essential steps in self-healing.

When you stop judging and criticizing yourself there's a release of tension. You feel more at ease within. Your confidence and self-esteem go up. Because you're no longer scrambling your attention through doubt and internal conflict, your mental, physical, and emotional energies naturally begin to gather. They start to work with, rather than against each other. This in turn contributes to a deeper feeling of overall well-being, and can result in the healing of many problems.

The Nature of Masculine and Feminine Energy

Something which can help you come to greater self-acceptance is to recognize that your energy tends to move, or manifest, in two primary ways. This is true of all of us, both men and women. No matter whether you're a man or a woman, you have elements of the opposite sex in your genes, your hormones, and your personality. Within you there is some of the energy of the opposite sex. These energies are referred to as "feminine" and "masculine." The ancient Chinese Taoists—followers of the *Tao*, the natural "way of life" philosophy espoused by Lao Tzu—called them *yin* for the former, and *yang* for the latter.

One of the key principles upon which Oriental medicine, including acupuncture, is based is the degree of balance between the *yin* and *yang* energies. Certain organs are characterized as having *yin* qualities, while others are said to be more *yang*. The different types of diseases are classified the same way, as are the appropriate treatments for them. The practitioner who understands the law of *yin* and *yang* aims to bring these two mutually interactive—but, just as in man-woman relationships, often conflictive—forces into a balanced whole.

If you're a man, then you have, in addition to your basic masculine energy, a feminine, or *yin* side to you. If you're a woman, you have a masculine, or *yang* side. Carl Jung, the Swiss psychiatrist who did so much to open up the realm of myth and symbol as it relates to the unconscious, called these same energies *anima*, for the feminine principle as it exists in men, and *animus* for the masculine principle in women.

The feminine principle is essentially non-active, receptive, nurturing. Very much present-time oriented, it is playful and spontaneous, concerned only with what is felt and experienced in the here-and-now. It delights in simply *being*—in being open to the beauty and the potential of the now moment. It's analogous to the right brain, which is the hemisphere that has been shown to be most responsible for intuition and imaginative, non-logical, non-directed thinking.

The masculine principle is more active, assertive, achievement-oriented. It is very linear, very directed. It doesn't like to just sit and *be*. Rather, it seeks out a goal, an objective, and moves toward it with calculated precision. It manifests in the activity of the left cerebral hemisphere, where the functions of reason and analytical thinking originate.

The feminine is warm and emotional. The masculine is cool and rational. The feminine relies on intuition, sees things holistically. It operates deductively, going from the general to the particular. The masculine is more intellectual, mathematical, and works through inductive reasoning. It forms conclusions and solves problems through accumulating separate chunks of information. The feminine is more concerned with *process*, simply experiencing and being open to whatever is happening. The masculine is concerned with *results*, with fixing, changing or doing something about what is happening.

Bringing the Two into Balance

If you are using both your intuition and your intellect as you read this, then you'll have already guessed (a feminine quality!)—or figured out (a masculine trait!)—that both modes of being have their value. To be a whole person, operating at your highest potential with all your resources available, you need to be in touch with both the feminine and masculine qualities within you. Instead of erring lopsidedly in one direction or the other—being excessively emotional and irrational, for example, or being so cerebral and "reasonable" that you're completely divorced from your feelings—the two polarities need to be brought into a healthy balance.

If you're a woman, you need to nurture your rational, linear, goal-oriented side in order to be whole. This means being able to stay focussed on an objective, without getting too emotionally involved in it. A certain detachment is required here. None of this is to be developed at the expense of your feminine qualities, but rather should complement them. Working a business, practicing martial arts, handling financial accounts, expository writing, debating, and learning to deal with confrontational situations from a position of strength and power are all opportunities for becoming more familiar with the classically masculine traits.

Men, on the other hand, learn about their feminine side through taking more time to just *be*, to enjoy non-goal-oriented activities such as play, and being in nature. Stopping to look at and smell the flowers, noticing the hills, gazing up at the sky and spending time in meditation, reverie, and daydreaming bring out the feminine qualities in men. Taking an active interest in parenting, in really being there for their children in a loving way, helps men who are fathers become more whole.

Honoring the feminine means giving more attention to relationships in general, learning to listen with an open mind and heart, without trying to "fix" the other person, without trying to solve problems. It's discovering that when you're truly present with another, attentive to that person without the need to say or do anything on your own part, miracles can sometimes happen.

When there is space for the other person to open up, often the simple act of sharing, of unburdening, brings about a healing. Very often, these kinds of interactions—without any evident purpose or direction, but taking place in an environment of warmth and affection—can be more satisfying, enriching, and enlightening than anything you might accomplish through a more active, forceful "doing."

Few things serve as a more powerful catalyst for healing than the realization that someone cares enough to listen, and to be there.

The Dominance of the Masculine

From a social perspective, the more "civilized" and technologically-oriented a society is, the more patriarchal, or masculine, it tends to be in its values. New technologies are developed based on scientific understanding, which stems from objective, linear, analytic thinking. It's termed "hard" data—an interesting choice of words when you consider that male scientists, technicians, and engineers can sometimes by very "hard" in their emotional relating.

Setting goals and working toward their accomplishment in a direct, logical, and methodical fashion is important in a patriarchal system. Success is measured by statistical results. Unlimited growth is of paramount importance, and having or achieving "more" of anything is judged to be better than settling for less.

The social advantages of these masculine values are self-evident. Technology provides us with the physical necessities and comforts we need in order to sustain an efficient, cost-effective lifestyle. It enables us to tap into the agricultural, geological, and other material resources necessary for food, clothing, shelter, and transport. It can take care of many repetitive, boring, or dehumanizing tasks that would otherwise have to be performed by human labor.

But the disadvantages and limitations are becoming equally obvious to us. Of what benefit is scientific and technological advancement if it isn't used with wisdom and a caring heart? What is the value, in human terms, of being a wealthy society if most of the wealth rests in the hands of a small section of the population, while too many continue to struggle along in poverty? Or if technology is used by the government in order to control and repress the common people, and to put down any attempts at dissent, at divergent or oppositional thinking? Or, as in the case of the United States, if a nation's medical care and standard of living is rated among the best in the world, yet there are more than twenty countries where the infant mortality rate is lower?

Learning from Traditional Societies

A nation can't be healthy unless the individuals who govern it are healthy. In our modern society, we've over-valued the patriarchal, masculine qualities that are the underpinnings of science and technology.

In more traditional, peasant-type societies the matriarchal, or feminine qualities, are not so repressed. Intuition and imagination are valued. Space and time take on a different meaning. People live much more in the present. They have a concerned, intimate relationship with the earth, with their physical environment. This is reflected in their art, their stories, and their legends. They look to and rely on the seasons. They care about the well-being of their environment. Rather than trying to control the outcome of events through intellect and will, they grow up learning to listen to and trust the wisdom and rhythms of nature.

Much can be learned from observing these more traditional societies. It's no accident that there is such a renewal of interest in them. An increasing number of people have become interested in learning about Native American ways. Until they were dispossessed by the Europeans who took over their lands, Native Americans lived in harmony with nature. They were a deeply spiritual people.

The popular Goddess movement is another example of the desire many people have to return to a more natural way of living. Many concerned women and men are beginning to discover the treasure of ancient knowledge handed down to us by the matriarchal tradition that dominated most of the earth's peoples, prior to the rise of the Judeo-Christian culture.

Healing Comes through the Feminine

Because of our social and cultural conditioning, most of us, especially men, tend to be ruled by the *yang*, or masculine energies. We've been conditioned to believe that it's the masculine qualities that make for material wealth and career success. And yet it's these very same qualities that are behind so much of the stress we endure. We feel constantly pushed to be more, have more, accomplish more. Accumulation is the name of the masculine game. But through all this frantic pursuit of an elusive happiness and fulfillment outside, inside the masculine soul there's a hunger and emptiness that won't go away.

If the real yearning inside us isn't acknowledged and satisfied, we suffer. This is our spiritual hunger, our deep human need to live an inspired, creative life. When the longing for spiritual fulfillment goes unheeded we harden, we become frustrated, we get sick from any number of increasingly prevalent stress-related diseases.

Sooner or later, however, if the longing gets acute enough, we wake up. We get wise. It dawns on us that the healing we're looking for can only come through the feminine, through bringing out the repressed or long dormant receptive, nurturing, creative side of ourselves. This is the lover, the meditator, the artist, the playful child within.

You may remember the lines I quoted in the chapter on movement from Stephen Mitchell's translation of the *Tao Te Ching*. The whole book is a hymn to the virtues of soft power, the feminine. It teaches that the soft will always overcome the hard, and that only in surrendering control do you find yourself at the center, the ground of all possibilities. Let me give you another verse, paraphrased from several sections in the book. I think it sums up, beautifully, the essence of this philosophy.

> *His body is supple as a newborn child's.*
> *His heart and mind open as the sky.*
> *Realizing that nothing is lacking,*
> *The whole world belongs to him.*
> *This is the Master's secret.*

In my work with people I am constantly reminded of the healing power of the feminine. I remember a woman patient who was going through a great deal of suffering, both physical and emotional. After working together for a few sessions, I couldn't help but notice how hard she was on herself, how critical, rejecting, and non-accepting of herself she was.

She had very strong feelings about many things, and felt guilty for having them. Her own self-judgment—learned, it became clear, from her parents when she was growing up—lay behind her guilt.

She'd come to believe she was a "bad" person. Her sense of self-worth, of self-esteem, was very low. She was always putting herself down, always talking about the futility of attempting anything new because it was almost a given, in her bitter experience, that she'd fail.

At one point I found myself wanting to say, "Hey, be a little easier on yourself!" Then I began to realize she'd lost touch with her own femininity, her own softness. Even the spiritual path she'd been on for many years was very masculine in its approach. It stressed intellectual understanding and emotional detachment, a linear progression toward some ideal of "enlightenment." Interestingly, her teacher was a man, and was known to be aloof, authoritarian, and patriarchal.

Working with this woman helped remind me of how vital a role the feminine energy plays in healing, and how essential is the need for compassion—for softness, gentleness, openness, patience. We need this not only in ourselves, but also in our mentors, those to whom we look for encouragement and guidance. Like so much in life, it's a paradox, because we also need the balance of the masculine. We need firmness as well, we need to know when to take a strong stand. We need to be able to commit ourselves decisively to a course of action when such commitment is required.

Learning to open to the feminine has been one of the key elements in my own healing. I've seen this time again with others. I know both men and women who, over the years, have been going through a genuine transformation. In each case it's always the same: the hard edges are disappearing, the ego is less shrill, there's a softening in the voice and the eyes, the heart is opening. They are more present, more human. It's a beautiful thing to witness, to see an old friend growing into this kind of richness and fullness of being.

Opening to the Feminine

More than anything, it's the ability to be sensitive to what we're feeling that characterizes the feminine aspect of ourselves. This is why the chapter on learning to trust what you're feeling is such an important thread in the overall fabric of this book. The cure for emotional suffering lies in opening to your feelings.

I remember how, years ago when I met Barbara, she continually asked me what I was feeling. I'd make what I thought was a perfectly reasonable response to her question, and she'd immediately shoot back with, "Yes, but what are you feeling?"

"What do you mean 'What am I *feeling*?'" I'd reply impatiently, for the truth was that in those days, I seldom really knew what I was feeling. My life was lived mainly in my head. Reason, logic, and intellectual wordplay were my gods. There was an explanation for everything, I believed, and if I couldn't immediately find one, then with my clever, calculating mind (a very masculine quality!) I could soon make one up.

But Barbara kept probing, so strong was her need for emotional contact with me. Intellectual concepts and brilliant theories didn't impress her. "What are you feeling?" she'd persist, and gradually, I gave way. I couldn't have done otherwise. Feelings are soft, fluid, melting. As the *Tao Te Ching* so eloquently says:

> *Nothing in the world*
> *is as soft and yielding as water.*
> *Yet for dissolving the hard and inflexible,*
> *nothing can surpass it.*

So I began to learn the language of feelings. It was a slow process. Like most men, I was very resistant to owning my feelings, much less talking about them. There were actually a lot of painful feelings inside me, feelings of resentment, fear, inadequacy. I'd developed my mind, had become something of a master at the fine art of rationalization, precisely so that I could distance myself from those feelings. I did all I could to avoid having to feel them.

But Barbara's soft, feminine power gradually melted down the hard masculine defenses I'd spent so many years shoring up. My ego began to release some of its grip on me. My heart began to open, and I started to feel myself more deeply. It became easier to talk about my inner condition, and I found it enormously freeing—even though it was threatening at first—to do so.

Reconciling the Two Energies

Eventually I began to work with some male teachers whose *yin* and *yang* energies were already in a healthy balance. These were men who were successful in their lives in the ordinary sense, the one that is so important to most men and that has to do with career and accomplishment. Yet they were genuinely *present* as human beings too. They had a warmth and sensitivity about them, as well as strength and power. They had their egos still, but they didn't let them prevent their hearts from being open. It felt surprisingly safe to be with them. Their willingness to be vulnerable made it easier for me to let my defenses down.

In time, I learned that whenever I felt myself contracting and hardening, it served me to remember to soften, to let go. I made a conscious practice of it. Even though I often resisted the women in my life, and the demands they made upon me for emotional connection, I eventually became grateful for their presence. They reminded me, through their simple femininity, of where the true healing lay.

Women, I realized, embodied the virtues of softness and warmth. They were generally more present than men. I had to admit that many of the women I knew were often closer to God, more in touch with their spirituality, than I was. Their ability to simply be in the moment, open to their feelings, gave them an ease that I lacked. They had fewer ego problems. For a man like myself, who had definite ideas about who he was and where he was going, being around a woman who insisted that he take a deeper look at himself and what he was feeling inside, was often intimidating. It meant having to confront my own rigidity, my masks and defenses—and behind them, my fear and insecurity.

Women, too, can forget their real nature and can sometimes be as hard and unyielding as any man. We all have the potential for hardening our hearts, just as we all have it within us to feel deep compassion and caring. As always, wholeness is found in the balance, in the reconciliation of the two energies within, the masculine and the feminine. It means a willingness to be present, to listen, to feel, to be vulnerable. It means having the strength to stand firm in our vulnerability, so that we don't run or hide when things get uncomfortable.

Finding that balance within yourself and learning to live with it in a world where conflict and competition are still the rule, where hardness is misperceived as strength, and vulnerability as weakness, is one of the more demanding pieces of healing work you'll do.

Yet it's essential. As you become more successful at integrating the two polarities, you'll experience less inner conflict. You'll feel more whole within, more fully yourself, and your relationships with others will be much more harmonious and satisfying.

Forgiveness, the letting go of blame, is the key to healing any relationship. That, and the realization that relationship begins at home. You can't have a happy relationship with someone else until you're at peace with yourself.

Chapter 13
Heal Your Relationships

Relationships are one of our most powerful teachers of what it means to be a whole human being. They are probably the best mirror you'll ever have for seeing yourself, for learning about both your strengths and your flaws, about what you do well and what you do poorly in life. Live with a man or woman—your spouse or partner—for a few years, and you'll get more than enough feedback as to what the other person likes and dislikes in you. Sometimes the feedback may be more candid than you'd rather hear!

It's relatively easy to feel serene and at peace when you're alone meditating in your favorite place, or taking a solitary walk in nature, or doing something else by yourself that you love to do. It's quite a different proposition finding that same serenity when you're living with another human being who may have a very different perspective on life than you do, and who frequently has different wants and needs.

What is the key, then, to healing the conflict that exists in so many relationships? How do you know when the healing has happened? These are some of the questions I'll address in this chapter. In some ways this may be one of the most important chapters of all in this book, because the proof that you're healing inwardly—emotionally and spiritually—shows in the ease with which you're able to be with and relate to others.

The way many people deal with conflict in their relationships is simply to avoid, wherever possible, those relationships. The problem with this approach is that if it really is an avoidance, a refusal to look at some emotional issue that is triggered by a particular relationship, then you don't grow. You never have the opportunity to heal that emotional wound within you. Without the healing, you're never going to actualize all of who you are. You are cutting yourself off from an essential part of yourself.

As you begin to address your emotional wounds, the energy behind them becomes more integrated. When you deny an aspect of yourself, however—such as a fear around commitment, or a fear of being abandoned—you're splitting your own energy. You're literally pushing a part of yourself down, repressing it, and this itself takes a lot of energy. To hold yourself back or deny yourself in this way can, over many years, result in a variety of stress-related illness and diseases, as well as frustration and unhappiness.

Healing the Wounds of the Past

It is in your relationships that you have the chance to heal these wounds. The hurts themselves date from your early childhood experiences, from your relationship with your parents. It has been said that you can't have a healthy, intimate relationship with another person until you have healed your relationship with your parents. I've found this to be true, though the healing doesn't necessarily take place in a linear fashion. It's not as if you can go back, heal your relationship with your parents and then, once you've gotten that all squared away, so to speak, proceed to have a conflict-free relationship with your partner. It doesn't happen quite that easily.

It helps, though, if you can take an honest look at the relationship you had—or have—with your parents. What was the communication like in your family? Were you encouraged to talk about your feelings and to express your needs? Did you feel supported, emotionally nourished, loved? Were your parents good role models for you? If they are alive now, do you enjoy being around them, or at least feel comfortable when you're with them? If they've passed away, are you at peace with your memories of them?

If you're like many people, you couldn't readily answer "Yes" to these questions. For many of us our relationship with our parents, when we look back at it, was at best unsatisfying. There may not have been a lot of negativity, but it wasn't necessarily a wholly positive experience either. For many other people, the experience of growing up was so painful that life has been extremely difficult for them ever since. The large numbers of people who spend year after year in therapy, dealing with the low self-esteem they acquired as a result of their unhappy childhood conditioning, is evidence enough of this.

Therapy can be of value in helping us heal those old wounds. The psychotherapeutic process has its limitations, however, especially if it focuses on dealing endlessly with every little trauma, or past hurt, that was ever sustained by us. Good therapy doesn't go on forever. What it will do is bring the kind of understanding that can facilitate movement in your life—as opposed to the "intellectual" understanding that just results in new beliefs and rationalizations, with no real change.

Boundaries

A good therapist will teach you about the importance of having healthy boundaries. John Bradshaw, who has done much to expand the public's awareness of the dynamics of dysfunctional families, has stated that relationship problems are primarily boundary problems. Either our boundaries tend to be too loose, which means we get emotionally and psychically enmeshed with others, or they are too rigid. When it's the latter, we keep others at a distance, never allowing them to get close to us—and so denying ourselves any opportunity for genuine intimacy.

In either case, the problem is fear and insecurity. The healing comes as we get to know ourselves better, and learn how to take a stand for what we believe in, for what we feel and need. People with weak boundaries need to learn to be strong and more self-contained, so that they can say "No" to those who tend to be invasive or emotionally-draining. People with too tightly-controlled boundaries, on the other hand, need to loosen up. They need to learn to say "Yes" to life, and to trust that they will be able to handle the intense feelings that come up when others start to get close to them.

Good therapy, wise counsel, can help us learn all this. The best counseling has a spiritual, or transpersonal, perspective to it. The transpersonal approach helps you build not only a healthier ego, or sense of personal identity, but it also helps you get in touch with who you are beyond your ego. It directs you back to the source of love within you, so that you're not always looking to someone else to fill the emptiness in your heart.

This is where the real healing lies. The more in touch you are with your spirituality, the clarity and wisdom within you, the less identified you are with the problems and conflicts in your life. You're not so reactive, because you have more perspective on the issues before you. You're able to see what needs to be done, and you're better equipped to muster the courage and resolve necessary for decisive action.

There is one thing of supreme importance for the healing of any relationship difficulty, whether it's with your parents, your lover or partner, your children, or someone else, such as a co-worker: you have to really *want* to heal it. This may sound obvious, yet this simple fact often eludes us. If you have a genuine desire to heal your relationship with your parents, for example, then in a very real sense, that's all that's required. Willingness is the first step in healing any relationship. When a desire is strong enough, a powerful creative energy is unleashed. That energy will draw to you the help and guidance needed to facilitate the healing.

Remember, too, that in the end it's only your own healing that you can directly influence. For example, if your parents are living and still, in your experience, emotionally contracted in their outlook and behavior, there may not be anything you can do about it. They just may not want to open up. If they are dead—and died angry, depressed, or unhappy—there is certainly nothing you can do to change the past.

But you can do something about your own inner process—and here we come to the heart of healing as it applies to all relationships. It's to be found in forgiveness. Forgiveness is the letting go of blame for all the past hurts and grievances the other persons may have caused you, and learning to accept them as they as, for who they are.

How does this acceptance show? It shows in the fundamental respect you begin to have for their beingness, their humanity. It shows in a willingness to overlook their personal faults, their negative traits. It shows in kindness and courtesy—and, when necessary, firmness—in your dealings with them. It shows in the expanded feeling of well-being you'll experience once you stop judging them. It shows in the sense of freedom you feel as you stop making them wrong for the way they've treated you in the past, or the way in which they may continue to treat you in the future.

No One is to Blame

I remember a time when a former partner and I were going through some intense conflict. It was the kind of power struggle that many couples come to, once the "honeymoon" period of the relationship is over. I was aware of feeling a lot of anger and resentment toward her. If someone had asked me, I could have readily checked off all the reasons why I was unhappy—and almost all of them because of her.

At the same time, I loved her, and I found these conflicting feelings of mine disconcerting. I realized that for my own peace of mind, as well as the health of our relationship, I needed to get some clarity. I needed some kind of resolution of the conflict within me before there could be a healing of the struggle between us. So I did what I've learned to do with really difficult personal problems like this: I brought the situation into my meditation.

I sat, took the time necessary to get quiet and still, and then allowed myself to open up to that spacious feeling which unfolds when we're really present. Soon I was aware of a deep silence, a healing energy of peace and tranquility. Yet when I acknowledged what was going on within me emotionally, there was still a residue of anger. There was no denying the anger, no escaping it, so I gave my attention to it. I allowed it to just be there, to grow a little and to begin to roil around inside me. It's an interesting and revealing process, this looking at a problem—and especially at one that is emotionally-charged—while in meditation.

When you're able to be present with a problem in this way (and it takes time and experience to get to this place where you can just *be* with it), the disturbance can be there, and yet it doesn't overtake you. You're aware of the disturbance, you're feeling it, but you're not so identified with it. Because you're connected to that larger energy, to spirit, you're able to maintain some perspective on your feelings and emotions.

There's a caution here, however. This process only works effectively when the pain or disturbance you're experiencing is already somewhat manageable. I'll go into this more thoroughly later, but when the pain is overwhelming, trying to come to terms with it in meditation is usually not an option. There's nothing to do but feel it. Later, when the emotional upheaval has subsided, you can sit with it on your meditation cushion.

During my meditation I allowed the feelings of anger and resentment, and the vague notions of all that I thought was "wrong" with my partner, to rise up into my consciousness. Everything became somewhat dark and began to coalesce into one heavy, wearisome mass. It was a very negative energy. It had a mesmeric quality to it. I started to feel physically tired, so that I began to lose my attentiveness. Contemplating my feelings around my relationship was starting to drag me down. I yawned. Maybe I should just forget about it, I thought. Maybe I should just lie down and go to sleep.

Then suddenly a bright and clear image floated up from some deep recess of my psyche. It was the cover of a book I'd read a long time ago, Bob Hoffman's *No One Is To Blame*. Instantly, I was alert again. The book's blue, green, and white cover—and especially the words, *No One Is To Blame*—hovered in my field of awareness. Then the image disappeared, and without my having to think or speculate about it, the meaning of what I'd seen flooded into my mind.

No wonder I was confused! I'd been blaming my partner all these years for the things I was unhappy about in our relationship. How could I begin to see anything clearly if I'd already made a decision that she was the one largely at fault? Hadn't she herself taught me long ago that piece of wisdom from Lao Tzu's *Tao Te Ching*, about "no fight, no blame?"

The message was undeniable. I wouldn't get any clarity about our relationship until I stopped blaming her. And the beauty of the whole revelation as it came to me during meditation was that, truly, no one was to blame! We had different needs, different wants, yes, and the conflict between us lay in our inability to find a common ground. But neither of us was to blame for the conflict.

In the days following that meditation, the effect of what had been given to me began to show itself spontaneously. I didn't have to "work" at not blaming her. Because I'd seen the truth—and because it had come not from my intellect, but from a place very deep inside me, a place that was connected to divine wisdom itself—I just naturally began blaming her less.

I may not have stopped doing it completely, but I could no longer do it and still feel good about it. Gradually, the pattern of blame began to fall away, and it shifted the dynamics of our relationship. This is the magic of consciousness. When one partner goes through a transformation like this, the other person cannot help but be affected by it.

When I stopped blaming her, I ceased giving her the ammunition she needed to blame me in return. We moved to a new level of understanding. We were able to more realistically talk about the problems between us.

Forgiveness

To truly let go of blame is enormously healing. It frees us from the painful effects of the past, and from the certainty of continued suffering in the future.

When we forgive someone who has hurt us—a parent, a lover, a friend—we release that person from our psyche, our energy field. No longer are they held there as a negative energy—a memory, an image—eating away at our well-being. As we let them go, we discover more of ourselves, our own authentic energy. "Forgiveness is the key to happiness," teaches the *Course In Miracles*. We begin to understand why. Forgiving is not so much an affirmative process, as in saying, "I forgive you," though there's a time and a place for this. Rather, it's a letting go of the blame and resentment you're holding onto. For forgiveness to happen, the other person need not even be alive. It's the negative memories about them that are the upsetting factor, and it's these that must be released.

Ironically, you don't even have to think about forgiving the other person. In fact, you're not even doing it for them, at least not initially. (As your compassion grows, you'll be more concerned with the welfare of others). You're doing it for *you*. To forgive is to let go of the attitudes and mindsets that are hurting *you*. How wonderful it feels to unburden yourself in this way!

Forgiveness is only difficult when you don't have a strong desire to heal yourself and be free. If you're more invested in staying angry or bitter, then all the techniques in the world for practicing forgiveness won't work. But when your desire to live a happy and peace-filled life becomes more important to you than continued emotional pain and suffering, then to stop blaming—and start forgiving—makes a whole lot of sense.

Being a Victim

The error we make in relationships, and the reason why they cause so much pain, is that we still so often cling to the illusion that we're at the effect of other people's behavior. We persist in believing that they somehow have control over our destiny. There was a certain amount of truth to this when we were children. Back then we were relatively powerless to take a stand for our own freedom. We hadn't yet undergone the ego development and the capacity for discrimination, for making wise choices, that come with maturity.

Fortunately, most of us are raising our children now far more consciously than we were raised. We're encouraging our children to express their needs and wants, to stand up for their own truth, to speak out when they feel they aren't being treated fairly by one or both parents. In a conscious family, children are not arbitrarily ruled over or dominated by their parents. They are *guided* by them. And the governing principle of this guidance is a respect for the children's right to be. It's an honoring of their right to be free, creative, and happy individuals.

Without this kind of intentional upbringing, however, our childhood conditioning usually results in feelings of powerlessness and victimhood. We grow up expecting to have boundaries and limits imposed on us by others. We seek the approval of others, believing we must have it before we can take action or accomplish anything. We don't have a vital connection to our own internal power. We don't have any real idea at all of our true capabilities or potential.

What results from growing up like this is the belief that we aren't enough by ourselves. We then move into adulthood convinced that we need a partner in our lives—a man or a woman—in order to make us whole. This conviction ran me for many years. Because I wasn't in touch with my own *anima*, the feminine principle within me—my feelings and emotions—I was always expecting a woman to complete me, to make my life whole. I relied on women for emotional nurturing and stimulation. Getting free of this reliance was a long and challenging process.

It wasn't until I was finally rejected by a woman I loved very much—a woman who saw my desperate need for her and ran, literally, in the other direction—that I was forced back on myself. I had to face the pain of rejection, of losing the person I thought I was going to be with for the rest of my life. The loss was the most emotionally-devastating experience I'd ever gone through. It shook me to my core, so much so that nothing I'd previously believed in—not even my spiritual beliefs—meant anything anymore.

In the past, it was I who had done the rejecting, I who had been the heart-breaker. Now, I was thrown into the darkest period of my life.

Facing the Pain of Rejection

When my lover left me, I didn't know what to do. I couldn't believe such a thing was happening to me. I thought we were friends. I thought we had a good thing together. How could I have been so blind as to not see what was really going on with her?

Even my attempts at meditation didn't ease the pain, so intense was my suffering. There was nothing I could do but feel all my feelings, cry all my tears—and, as clarity gradually began to dawn, to see that what I'd been in love with was, to a very large degree, an illusion of my own making. I'd idealized this woman. I'd made her into something she wasn't—the "perfect" image of the one who was going to bring me lasting happiness. At some level my lover had sensed all this, and it was partly why she left. She could no longer fulfill my need for her to be the Goddess in my life. She just wanted to be herself.

Once she was gone, I was left totally on my own. She'd brought an enormous amount of light into my life, a depth of beauty, passion, and joy that I'd never before experienced with such consistency. Now, I realized, I had to find the light within me again. I saw that I had to let go of the illusions, the images, the fantasy I'd built up around who she was and what she meant to me. In letting go of the "story" I'd made up around her that had become, literally, an obsession, I slowly came back to something authentic within me.

At first I felt achingly alone and empty. My life seemed dark, futile, meaningless. But as I allowed myself to have my feelings, to experience my grief, the emptiness began to turn to fullness. My heart was open, flowing with feeling. As painful as that period of my life was, I certainly felt very *alive*.

Gradually, I began to find my own light again. It became easier to meditate, to consciously see her with more compassion, and to let her go. It helped me to realize that it wasn't my fault that she'd left. Our time together was over. She was just following the call of her soul. The cherished images of her began to fade as I took up the broken threads of my life, and got back into my work, my creativity, and my relationship with my son—all of which had been neglected, so caught up was I in my own suffering.

The Path of the Heart

Losing what I thought was the best relationship I'd ever had was one of the major turning points in my life. It brought a new meaning to my understanding of spirituality, and what it meant to be a whole person. It shifted me out of my intellect—the philosophical "bubble" I'd lived in for so many years—and brought me more fully into my heart.

Before, my spirituality was always somewhat detached and aloof. I was most at peace sitting on my meditation cushion. I thought meditation would solve everything. I used to believe that if we'd all just meditate and find inner peace, everything would be okay. But the experience of being abandoned by my lover dislodged me from the comfort of my meditative refuge, and dumped me hard on the ground of reality. I could no longer avoid my feelings and emotions by escaping into the rarefied mental states induced by meditation.

In Buddhism, enlightenment has two complementary attributes: wisdom and compassion. Without compassion, wisdom is detached, cold, unfeeling. Without wisdom, compassion drifts all too easily into helpless emotion and pity. Through meditation and self-inquiry, I'd gained some wisdom. Now, with this experience of suffering, I was getting an important lesson in compassion. My heart was opening. Instead of trying to tell people how to transcend their suffering, I was beginning to have more empathy for what they were going through. I could relate to the pain they were feeling, because I was feeling the same pain myself. It was almost as if I could hear God saying to me, "Welcome to the human race, Jim."

It's a bitter irony that, so often, the heart must be broken before it can really open. When we're young, our hearts are naturally open. As we grow up, the emotional pain and trauma we experience causes us to close down, to build a shell around our hearts. Healing at the emotional level challenges us to soften, to eventually break away that shell. It calls upon us to open to our feelings—and, especially, to the feeling of compassion, compassion for both ourselves and for others.

As in the practice of homeopathy, the cure often lies in the disease itself. It's usually only pain itself that initiates the opening that is so sorely needed if we're to be emotionally healthy. Pain can initiate very deep healing. So long as we feel content, satisfied with the way things are, we're not likely to want to change. But searing pain demands that we change. If we don't, we just close down even further, which only results in more suppression, with all its tragic consequences. Sadly, some choose to follow this latter path, and their lives become increasingly contracted and unhappy.

Dr. Naomi Rachel Remen, a holistic medical doctor from California, had this to say about the heart and healing, in an article in *Healing Currents: The Journal Of The Whole Health Institute* (Spring 1991):

"There is a general lack of meaning and purpose and significance that seems to underlie illness. What we call stress might really be spiritual isolation... What is spiritual isolation? Basically to me it seems that it's living with a closed heart... A cardiologist once said to me that the most popular surgery in this country, coronary by-pass surgery, is probably a metaphor. The problem with our culture is that we have by-passed the heart, especially in men. And we keep acting that out, over and over again in the operating room."

Dr. Remen adds, "It's very interesting how often the process of physical healing runs concurrently with the healing of the heart."

Opening the heart requires that the ego, self-will, be put aside. More than anything, it is the ego—"I *demand* this!"—that obstructs the flow of love, of real communication between two people. It is the ego's willfulness that separates people, destroys relationships, and breaks up friendships. The more you can get your own willfulness out of the way, the more space you allow for the other person to see how their self-will may be a factor in preventing the two of you from meeting.

Learning to live from your heart, from sensitivity, feeling, and intuition, brings you more into the present moment. To get to this place, the self-righteousness of the ego—and all the emotions breathing life into it—has to be relinquished. The ego doesn't live in the present. It's preoccupied with time, with the past and the future, and with its own survival.

A relationship may survive when your ego is still in control, but it won't flourish. For that to happen, you must listen to what your heart is saying.

Expressing Anger

If you feel yourself to be a victim in a relationship, the first step in getting free is to acknowledge the fact of how you feel. This is to move out of denial. It's to be truthful about the way things are. Telling the truth in this way is itself freeing. Once you face the truth of something, energy that was previously going into denial is liberated. You feel better about yourself now that you're no longer trying to escape the facts, and the new energy will help you move in a more positive direction.

The next step is the one we've already looked at, and that's to begin the process of forgiving the other person, the one who is making you feel such a victim. But first you have to work through your anger toward him or her. You can't get free of something if you haven't yet accepted it, if you're still in denial about it.

Find a healthy, appropriate way to express your anger and resentment. Bob Hoffman has the people he works with do "bitch" sessions around Mom and Dad, because it's our parents' negative emotional patterns that are the primary influence behind our own. Many therapists encourage their clients to work out their anger by beating a pillow with an old tennis racket, or with their fists. Sometimes they take it out on a telephone book with a rubber hose. Even screaming out your frustration in the car, or on an isolated beach or hillside, helps. Do whatever you need to do to let those strong feelings blow through.

Some people don't find it necessary to act out their anger in this way. Just to acknowledge that they have it, and to be able to sit with it and give it space to defuse itself—during meditation, for instance—is sometimes all that's needed. It requires considerable clarity and maturity to be able to do this, however, because there's always the risk of getting trapped in denial again. The mistake many meditators make is that they learn to "transcend" their uncomfortable feelings and emotions, without ever really dealing with them. When the meditation is over, the negative feelings soon re-emerge.

Another useful tool is to write a letter to the person you're angry at. Pour out all your feelings. Express all your rage, your hatred. Call him or her names if you must. Don't censor yourself. This is a therapeutic process, and the more uninhibited you can be in venting your upset, the more benefit you'll get from the exercise. Don't, however, mail the letter! If you do, you'll just make the other person even more defensive. They'll get angry at you, and the relationship will degenerate even further. This is something you're doing for yourself. When all your anger is written out, read the letter as many times as you need, then put a match to it. Make the burning itself a ritual. Let the fire of your anger be transformed by the flames dancing before you.

Whatever your approach, there'll come a time when you'll realize that your anger doesn't have the same charge behind it. You may find yourself more in touch with your pain, your original hurt. Underneath anger, there is always pain—the pain of being discounted or ignored, or being insulted or attacked.

Feel your grief. Let the waves of emotion come, and then subside again. This is the beginning of the letting-go process. You're giving your real feelings space to express themselves. You've stopped blaming the other person, which is to direct your attention outward, and you've brought your attention back to what's actually going on inside you. You've taken responsibility for your own feelings. This results in a depth of healing that can never happen as long as you're pointing the finger and blaming.

You start to feel lighter. Forgiveness then follows naturally. Letting go of all the energy you were holding around the other person often has a positive and unexpected effect. You may find that person's attitude toward you changing, softening. He or she is no longer so defensive toward you.

Sometimes nothing will happen, the other person won't change at all. He or she may continue to avoid you, or still try to confront you. If this happens, it's because that person is not yet ready to heal the relationship. The person isn't yet ready to forgive, to let go. But at least you're no longer caught in blame.

Finding Harmony

Once there is forgiveness on both sides of a relationship, then there's space for the two of you to go deeper, if you wish. This is where a relationship between two people can lead to real intimacy. When you share a deep connection with another human being, a joining of the heart, mind and spirit, it can be a beautiful and enriching experience. You become a team. You're on each other's side. When two people are genuinely in tune with each other, energy multiplies and there are few limits to what you can create together.

Such limits as you do impose on your relationship will depend on the form of your relationship. A marriage or live-in relationship has the potential for a broader range of possibilities than a simple friendship. However, you may find that you can't share certain aspects of yourself with your partner because of the risk of hurt feelings. Some people just don't want to hear every truth. You may have a friend in your life then, someone with whom you can share this side of yourself because your friend is much more accepting of who you are. That person doesn't, after all, have to live with you!

Consider yourself fortunate if you have a partner who reflects all the different aspects of yourself, so that all your relationship needs are being met. It's not often that we find it all in one person—the honesty, the emotional nourishment, the intellectual stimulation, the sexual fulfillment, the play and laughter, the compatible financial values, the shared goals and vision, and the spiritual connection. While it's a blessing when we do have all that in one relationship, for most of us it remains something to be worked toward.

What makes it difficult to create true wholeness in a relationship is that it has to be a *shared* goal. You both have to feel strongly about connecting on every level. You both have to want it. There has to be a mutual willingness. If you each want something different it's hard to create a harmonious dance together.

Many couples have different interests, things they like to do apart from each other, but they share a real desire to be with each other and a common vision for their future. The vision may be to attain financial security, to raise a family, or to grow old together, looking after and nurturing each other. Or—and I believe this is the highest form of relationships—it may be the recognition that the two of you are soulmates, and are meant to be with each other, to grow deeper in spirit.

Getting clear about what each of you wants separately, and then together, is an important relationship agenda. It's necessary to do this if you wish to travel far on the couple's journey. Otherwise you'll always be at odds. So you have to be clear about what you want. You have to be frank about what is important to each of you, what your actual relationship needs are.

Jean Klein said once, in response to a question about the art of having a happy marriage, "You must choose someone whose attributes are harmonious with your own." This is excellent counsel, but it presupposes that you're starting out relatively free of your past baggage and that you're choosing consciously—from clarity, from openness, from an intelligent awareness of what is in your own and the other's best interests.

Bringing the Unconscious Patterns into Consciousness

Most of us don't come into new relationships with the kind of clean emotional sheet that allows for conscious choices. Often, the unconscious factors play as big a role as the conscious attraction. We don't realize it at the time, but our soul is pulling us toward the other person because we have lessons to learn. We have vital developmental steps to complete, and it's through our relationships that we complete them.

For example, a man who is very cerebral and withheld emotionally, may find himself attracted to a woman who expresses her feelings and emotions with unbounded passion. Both parties may recognize areas of incompatibility between them. One or the other may sense, at the outset, that there's something not quite right in the match. There's something amiss that one or both knows is going to be a problem, yet the inconsistency is overlooked. Each has what the other needs most at the time. The woman can teach the man how to soften his rigidity and open to his feelings. The man can teach the woman more self-control and independence. Neither party is aware of it at the time, but their souls' desire for learning, for self-actualization, becomes the driving force behind the relationship

So the relationship begins, and the learning gets underway. The couple may do their dance for years—laughing, crying, fighting, playing, demanding, withdrawing, doing all the things that couples do when they're forever "working on" their relationship. Yet sooner or later the smoke clears. The major lessons have been learned, and the problems that were there at the beginning of the relationship, the things that were never really quite right, become increasingly evident.

Some couples manage to work through these problems, or at least come to a degree of acceptance around them. They continue to live together, some genuinely learning to love, others satisfied with being reasonably content. But one person may be unwilling to settle for "reasonably" content. He or she may want more. Perhaps one of the parties can't tolerate the lack of harmony any longer, and feels the need to leave. Perhaps one person has grown in ways the other hasn't. Now that that person knows—or intuits—what's possible in a relationship, he or she would rather be alone than continue to live in an unfulfilling relationship.

Many of us, it seems, need to go through a number of long-term relationships in order to undertand what we need in a mate or partner. It's always sad when we end a relationship, especially when there are children involved in the break-up, yet sometimes it's the wisest thing to do. Sticking it out for the sake of the kids, the marriage vows, or anything else may only lead to further pain. When our heart is not in the relationship the other people feel it, and they suffer too.

So long as we're truly following our heart, the negative fall-out of leaving a relationship is minimized. We may move on physically from a relationship, but it needn't diminish the caring or the love we feel for those we've left behind. Perhaps we can love them more fully, more unconditionally, now that we no longer live with them. At last we may able to be a friend to them—and friendship is the foundation of any worthwhile relationship. Perhaps, by taking our own needed space, we have freed them to discover their autonomy, their strength, their own inner wholeness.

Relationships would be much easier if we started out with a strong sense of our own innate beauty and wholeness, but this rarely happens. We come into them with all our emotional baggage, the legacy of our past. The value of approaching our relationships as an opportunity for growth and learning is that it can help us heal the wounds we carry within us. It can help us mature. With each new stage of the relationship, each new phase of the power struggle, each new crisis and its resolution, we become—if we're awake to the opportunities before us—better and more whole human beings.

Relationship is fundamentally an inside job. To have the kind of clarity needed to make wise relationship choices, you have to know yourself well. You have to understand yourself, your needs and values, at a heartfelt level. The irony is that this kind of self-knowing—learning to bring the unconscious patterns into consciousness—usually only happens when we're in a relationship.

It gives a new twist to the old saying that you can't live with them, and you can't live without them!

Learning to Communicate Your Truth

One of the main stumbling blocks in relationships, whether it be a marriage, a friendship, or a business relationship, is the hidden agenda that get in the way of clear communication—the unacknowledged expectations, the withheld anger, the ulterior motives.

The truth can be threatening to our ego's sense of security. Much of the time we'd rather not hear it, nor speak it, because of the discomfort and pain it might bring up. So, fearing rejection, not wanting to be hurt—or to hurt—we refrain from expressing our real needs. We don't say what we feel. The sad consequence of this is that we live with the knowledge that something is amiss in the relationship. Something doesn't feel right, and nobody wants to talk about it.

The root meaning of the word communicate is "to share." For true intimacy to develop, you and your partner have to be able to share yourselves with each other. To feel safe to share, there has to be a basic acceptance of each other. This gives you the freedom in which to tell the truth. You can trust that the other person isn't going to jump all over you.

An effective exercise for improving the communication between you and your mate is to take some time as often as possible to just sit down and really be with each other. Twenty to thirty minutes is a good length of time for this exercise, which you might think of as a relationship "meditation." I first learned of it from a book called *Fire In The Heart: Everyday Life As Spiritual Practice*, by Roger Housden, an English author.

In this meditation, you sit opposite each other and connect by making eye contact and holding hands. Then you withdraw your

hands, and one person goes first. The person going first si[ ]
from their heart, about whatever they want to say.

You can view this as a clearing process, an opportunity [ ]
all the withheld communications, to speak of your hopes, needs, fears,
of anything that has been bothering you. It's your time to express anything you've been meaning or wanting to say to your mate. During this
exercise it's very important to make only "I" statements, to not get
into making "you" statements, other than in the context of how you
feel about something your mate may have said or done.

This is a "clearing" session, not a "dumping" session. You're
not to blame, criticize, or make the other person wrong. You're only
to speak of your experience. An example of such a statement might
be this: "When you yelled at me yesterday, I found myself getting
really upset, and I just wanted to storm out of the house." Putting it
this way permits you to state the truth of your own feelings, without
attacking your partner.

Throughout this exercise the other person just listens, without
any interruption. The partner who is playing the listening role
doesn't say a word. Restraint is paramount here. At the end of ten
minutes, or half-way through the time allotted for the session, you
both take time to be quiet, to center, and to make contact again
through the hands and eyes. The listener thanks the speaker for
sharing. Then it's the listener's turn to speak. That person, too,
speaks from their heart. (It's important for whoever is speaking second to remember that the goal is to simply share their truth, and not
get caught up in addressing or responding to what was said by the
other person.)

When a couple makes a commitment to doing this relationship
meditation on a regular basis, some very beautiful things can begin
to happen. First of all, because there is now structured time and
space for the sharing of truth, there is a deepening of intimacy.
You're practicing the art of giving your unconditional attention to
one another—perhaps the most important gift we can give anyone.

You're getting to know each other. Each of you has an opportunity to be heard, without being provoked or invalidated. If you're
both accustomed to meditating alone, then bringing this meditative
quality into your relationship can be very powerful. In the quiet

between your shared words, you'll begin to sense a deeper energy moving, the energy of spirit itself.

If you make this commitment to being truthful with each other, then in those moments when the communication between you breaks down—as it almost inevitably will!—the disruption need not be a major problem. You'll be able to see more clearly how such break-downs happen because of the intrusion of self-will.

You'll have the opportunity to choose again to get your ego out of the way, and to come back into your heart, into what you're actually feeling. Instead of focusing on the willful statements or words, you can share the real feelings behind them. Only when you put your ego aside can you be open and vulnerable in this way with your partner.

The growing intimacy between you, in turn, leads to greater acceptance of each other. The truth sets you free, and the best relationships are those where you can be truthful and honest, where you can genuinely be yourself. As Jean Klein has so wisely said, "We love most those around whom we feel the freest to be ourselves."

Doing this relationship meditation with your lover, or your partner, will renew and deepen the feelings of love and attraction that first drew you together. It will take you beyond what most of us normally think of as "love"—with all its notions of ownership and possession—into something that is beautiful and mysterious, and bigger than both of you.

Relationship Begins at Home

Getting to this depth of communication with someone else only happens as you find it within yourself. Relationship begins at home. Acceptance begins at home. You can't expect integrity, passion, wisdom, humor, creativity, and commitment from another person until you've begun to actualize those qualities within yourself. You may find them in your partner, but unless you're able to reciprocate them, it's unlikely your partner will keep opening up to you so fully. No one wants to keep giving out energy without receiving something in return. To do so is to end up being constantly drained.

At the same time, it's hard to share your truth with your mate unless you know what your truth is. You can't talk about your feelings if you're not yet in touch with them yourself. As you learn to bring out these qualities within you, you'll find that you don't have to work so hard at creating meaningful relationships with others. Things will tend to happen on their own.

The more you give yourself permission to be who you really are, the more you'll attract people who are equally committed to truth and authenticity. Those who aren't on the same path, who are more concerned with protecting their egos than relating from their hearts, will tend to drop out of your life. This is the law of attraction at work. Whatever it is we're working with, we seem naturally to attract others who are dealing with the same issues—and to repel those who aren't on the same wave-length.

I remember when I was dating a woman I really liked and I found myself falling into an old pattern. I started to say something that wasn't true in order to avoid what I thought was going to be an upsetting situation.

But I caught myself. I saw what I was doing, and I wasn't about to revert to that old, self-defeating behavior. I'd worked too long and hard to get free of it. I said to myself, "Jim, it doesn't matter how much you like this woman. If you can't be yourself with her, you don't want to be with her." So I came back to what was true. I shared my insight with her. Because she was as interested in the truth as I was, she appreciated my honesty, and it led to a new level of intimacy between us.

As you trust yourself to be more honest, you'll be less afraid to take emotional risks. You'll be more able to deal with any rejection that may come—whether from your lover, a friend, or from someone else in your life. Rejection won't crush you as it once may have done. You know your own boundaries, what you will and will not stand for, and it'll be easier for you to respect the needs and wishes of others.

You have yourself, this strong and loving "you" you're beginning to discover, and this is the most important relationship you'll ever have. Then you can handle it when someone says "No" to you. By the same token, it becomes easier to say "No"—and, equally, "Yes!"—to others.

Moments of Genuine Meeting

You begin to see that it's the quality of the contact with the other person that makes a relationship worthwhile, not the quantity of time you may spend together. Sometimes all it takes is a glance, a fleeting touch. You catch each other in an unguarded moment and perhaps for the first time ever, you really meet. Such moments of contact can make up for years and years of never really connecting, other than in the most superficial way.

I remember this happening with my father a couple of years ago. I was back in New Zealand, my country of birth, visiting family and friends. We were at dinner with my father and his wife. Dad and I'd always had a friendly relationship, had always been relatively at ease with each other. I'd never felt disapproved of or criticized by him. Still, there were occasions when I often found myself longing for a deeper relationship with him, for a more intimate connection. Sometimes I felt as if we were only touching the surface of what a father-son relationship could be.

We hadn't seen each other in five years, so the dinner was something of a celebration. We chatted as we ate our meal, catching up on what had been happening in the intervening years. Barbara was present, and our five-year-old son, Adam. Then, at one point during the conversation, Dad put down his knife and fork and turned in my direction. I stopped eating and turned to face him. There was a moment of silence. We just looked at each other. His eyes were bright, open. He was totally there.

As I looked into his eyes, I really saw him. I saw his essence, and I knew he was seeing mine. It was as if our souls embraced. We had known each other for more than forty years, and now we were finally seeing each other for the very first time. Not only did we see each other, but we liked what we saw. He gave an approving nod, and we both grinned. The dining room seemed to fill with light and love. The others realized something was going on, and stopped talking momentarily. But nothing needed to be said between the two of us. Truly, as Ramana Maharshi, the Indian sage, once remarked, "When heart speaks to heart, what is there to say?" Dad and I smiled at the others, then picked up our knives and forks and resumed eating.

That evening made me feel very happy about my relationship with my father. I felt complete with him. If he were to die or something else were to happen and I was never to see him again, it would have been all right. We had met in the deepest and most intimate way two human beings can meet—heart to heart, being to being.

Such moments of contact satisfy so deeply, so fully, that they can literally last us a lifetime. Of course Dad and I have met again, and there's something new in our relationship now. It's as if we now understand each other in the most fundamental way, and that has freed us both to simply enjoy the connection we have, without having to try to make anything special of it.

Relationships as a Spiritual Process

Even an unsatisfying, conflict-ridden relationship has something to teach us. Look carefully, and it will show you the ways in which it is difficult for you to be present, to really meet another person. The beautiful thing about all our relationships is that they bring out everything within us, both the best and the worst. This is why they are so spiritually empowering. Most of us need the mirror of another person in order to see ourselves clearly. The feedback we receive in our relationships is one of the most compelling teachers we'll ever have.

Welcome what is happening in your relationships then, even though it may, at this stage of your development, be causing you conflict or pain. Your relationships are one of the most accurate barometers available for showing you how well you're doing in your life. They help you peg exactly where you are, and what you need to work on.

If a relationship is not happy—whether at home, at work, or elsewhere—it almost always points back to something you need to look at in yourself. Maybe you need to make some changes in the way you relate. Maybe you need to listen more carefully—perhaps to the other person, certainly to your own inner truth. Maybe the lesson is that the relationship you're in just doesn't have any juice in it any more, and it's time to end it, or move it in another direction.

As you find more of yourself through examining how you conduct your life and your relationships, you'll begin to tap a deeper energy of joy and fulfillment within you, an energy that won't depend on someone else's acknowledgement or approval. Increasingly it will be your own experience, something no one else can take from you.

Then, like Chloe Goodchild, writing in her partner, Roger Housden's book, you'll be able to say to your mate, or your closest friend, "The experience of my own aloneness is fundamental to my appreciating our shared existence together... The more we both stand in the ground of our own Being, the more we can be a support to each other. It's a two-way process."

Then you'll understand the abiding truth about relationship: that it is above all a spiritual process, an act of communion. Relationships become genuinely loving as you each get beyond your egos—your separate, willful selves. When this begins to happen, you'll experience, firsthand, the beauty and power behind Jesus' saying, "Where two or three are gathered together in my name, there am I in the midst of them."

In such a relationship you have the greatest joy of all, the joy that is shared and that keeps on expanding.

There will always be problems. The way to deal with them is to not be so personally identified with them, but to just take care of them. Then the problems of living won't get in the way of your real purpose in life.

Chapter 14

See Problems as Opportunities

Behind our pursuit of such forms of transformational work as healing, psychotherapy, personal growth training, and the many spiritual practices that are available to us, lies our deep inner desire for freedom.

Consciously or unconsciously, we long to be free—free of conflict, fear, and insecurity, free from psychological and emotional suffering. We desire physical health, peace of mind, harmonious relationships, and the freedom to be ourselves, to express our creative energy in a way that is meaningful to us and of value to others.

And we yearn, too, most of us, for that sense of inner well-being, of spiritual unity and fullness, that we associate with the return to God, or the Source. This is the healing that we most deeply seek, the "ultimate cure" that is the theme of this book. When God, or spirit, or Buddha-nature—the clear, awakened state—is a reality for us, even if only for a few moments here and there, we're renewed, reborn, made whole again.

One of the common illusions that prevents us from moving closer to the freedom and fulfillment we seek is the notion that it will bring an end to all our problems. In fact we often define freedom, whether we perceive it as "spiritual" freedom, or merely "personal" freedom, as a freedom from problems. I remember that when I began my own spiritual journey many years ago I was convinced that if I could just get enlightened enough I'd be free, finally, of all worldly problems.

It took me a long time, and much conflict and suffering, before it began to dawn on me that even with enlightenment (which is not, I discovered, a final "end-point," but rather an ever-deepening and expanding state of awareness, openness, and humility), the problems do not go away. They just get easier to address, to take care of, because you're no longer so identified with them.

Once your security and well-being start to come from an inner spiritual source, rather than from conditions and circumstances out-side yourself, you don't take the problems of living as seriously any more. You don't depend on their outcome for how you feel about yourself. Your self-esteem is not tied to your bank account, your professional or social standing, or how successful you are in your marriage or family life.

It comes from within you, from a deep and abiding sense of your own innate wholeness and your connectedness to something larger in life, to the beauty of creation itself.

A Problem is Simply an Unattended Situation

But problems are still there, and and always will be. So long as you're alive in a physical body, there will be problems. They are an inherent aspect of the daily drama of living. They come with the territory, so to speak. The word problem derives from a Greek root meaning, "to lay before." A problem, then, is a situation that is "laid before" you. It's something that needs your attention.

The Sufis, the Islamic mystics who have so much to teach us about the joy of discovering God, the Beloved, while dwelling fully in the world, say that a problem is simply an unattended situation.

Take care of the situation, and you've taken care of the problem. It's learning to adopt a "No problem!" kind of attitude. You stay on top of things—which is another way of saying that you remain present, conscious, attuned to the need at hand—and handle problems as they arise, without fussing or complaining.

Your body, your relationships, your work, and your finances, for example, are areas of your life that will inevitably require some form of ongoing attention, or care, on a consistent basis, otherwise they are likely to fall into a decline. They'll almost certainly become a *problem*—an irritation, a source of conflict—if you fail to watch over them.

Science teaches us that the physical universe, the material world, is in a state of entropy, or disintegration. Everything is "running down." If you're over the age of forty, you only have to look at your own body to realize this. All living things grow old and die, and all material or physical objects sooner or later wear out.

Taking care of what you've accepted responsibility for—which includes your body, the relationships you've invested time and energy in, and your financial obligations—helps slow down and minimize the disintegration process, and keeps everything running at an optimal level.

Indeed, if you give enough love and attention to these things, the rewards can be gratifying, so that right up to the very end there is no sense of loss, only gain. Even though you'll grow old and your life will go through many cycles and changes, your fundamental experience becomes one of continuing rebirth and renewal. You grow into wholeness. You open up to a fuller and richer experience of *living*.

An Opportunity for Growth and Empowerment

Seeing problems in this way, as opportunities for growth and for maintaining a high degree of well-being, is itself healing. Each time you solve a problem there's the satisfaction of accomplishment, of having achieved something. You feel more confident about your abilities, more secure within. You realize, "Ah, I can do it. I'm equal to the challenge."

Learning to successfully handle the problems of everyday living, especially if you do it on a consistent basis, is empowering. You can see this with children who are taught to take responsibility for their problems, who are encouraged to believe that they are capable of dealing with whatever comes their way. Such children don't suffer from the self-doubt and low self-esteem that affects children who never receive this kind of loving guidance.

Many problems, of course, need never arise, but do so because of ignorance, inattention, or procrastination, waiting too long to deal with a situation that has gotten out of hand. Problems happen in relationships, for instance, when there is a failure of communication between you and your partner, when you take each other too much for granted, or when underlying dissatisfactions or resentments are allowed to build to the point where the tension becomes such that something has to give. Or your work can become a problem when your heart is not in it and yet you keep on doing it, trying vainly to convince yourself that it's worth the effort. This kind of attitude sooner or later leads to burn-out.

No matter how much you persist at an endeavor, if your heart isn't in it, you'll never be happy. And if you know you're not going to be truly happy or satisfied as a result of what you do, you won't allow yourself to succeed at it. You'll find some way to sabotage yourself—and that will create a whole new set of problems.

Sometimes the problems laid before you will seem insoluble. It may be that a job or relationship is simply no longer working for you. You've gone as far as you can with it. To continue with it, to try and keep it alive when there is really no more energy there, would only be self-defeating.

At such times the only solution to a problem like this may be to leave, even though to do so can be very painful—even scary, because of the uncertainty of the future. When these feelings come up it can help to remember that if a job or relationship isn't working for you, it's probably not working for the other person—or people—involved either.

Running Away Solves Nothing

Leaving is not always the answer. Very often you end up just trading one unsatisfying situation for another. This is especially so if you don't yet really know yourself deeply, if you're still confused about who you are and what you want in your life. When leaving is a running away, a reaction to something you don't understand or can't control, you risk getting trapped all over again.

You may find yourself excited by the prospect of a new job or relationship, but after you've been in it for a while the new situation starts to sour too. Sooner or later all your unresolved issues—your guilt, your doubts and anxieties, your fears around commitment and intimacy, your reluctance to confront the truth—surface. You take yourself—and all your emotional baggage—wherever you go. The issues you've been grappling with for so many years are still there, waiting to be dealt with. Your emotional and behavioral patterns, until they are understood and accepted, tend to act themselves out over and over again. Your problems don't magically go away.

How then, do you begin to liberate yourself from the kind of conflict and inner struggle that is behind so many of the worldly problems that make up human experience? It requires, as a first step, a genuine desire for freedom, for what Abraham Maslow termed "self-actualization." As I said in the previous chapter about healing your relationships, you have to really *want* it. It has to be more important to you than being safe and comfortable. Many of us find it all too easy to get caught in a rut. We like the familiar, we don't particularly like being disturbed. So we compromise, we trade off, we put up with situations which, if we were really in touch with our true Self, our spiritual nature, we'd find intolerable.

In the language of addiction and recovery, this kind of trade-off is called denial, a subject which we've already explored. Denial, the refusal to acknowledge the truth of something, is one of the main mechanisms the ego uses to defend itself. The ego fears its own anni-hilation and will do anything—including tell lies to itself—to ensure the survival of the beliefs and images that make up its identity.

The possibility of real change begins to open up for us only when we start to move out of denial. This means taking an honest look at yourself and your problems and saying, in effect, "Hey, this is not working for me any longer. Time is running out and I want to do something with my life. I want to find out who I am. I want to live." Sometimes, to get to this place, we'll even create a crisis—such as an accident, an illness, a divorce, a bankruptcy—to shock us into wakefulness and get our energy moving.

The second step is to realize that you find freedom through being fully in life and dealing with the problems that you have, not running away from them. This is a challenge that many truth-seekers have to face—the age-old conflict between the seemingly contradictory worlds of spirit and matter. The more you open up to your spiritual nature, the more reluctant you may be, at times, to deal with such mundane issues as exercising your body, working to pay the rent, or confronting the emotional issues that inevitably come up in relationships.

Yet you have to heal this split if you're going to live in the world without fear, as a whole human being.

How the Mind Creates Problems

The healing comes about as you realize that any split you feel between body and spirit is a contradiction that exists primarily in your mind, in your attachment to your beliefs and concepts about the way things are, or ought to be.

It's seeing that the mind, by its very nature, labels, judges, and divides one experience from another. In this way it actually *creates* problems. The mind thrives on duality, opposition, conflict—on making up and solving problems. It's like a game to the mind. Having problems, things to worry and obsess about, keeps it busy and gives it a reason for existing. The mind feeds on problems. So long as it has something to worry about, it ensures its own survival, its dominance.

Once you begin to see that duality, or conflict, is an inherent aspect of the mind, you start to understand why people who follow a religion but have not found true spirituality are forever arguing and fighting with each other. They don't have a direct, heartfelt experience of God, or spirit, but only their beliefs and ideas about it. When two differing beliefs meet, whether in the mind of one person or in the opposing minds of two, they clash. They create doubt in the one, and disagreement between the two. So long as you live from your mind—from thinking alone—you'll never know any real peace.

Modern physics and the great mystical traditions have shown us that reality is in fact a dynamic, interconnected whole, a continuum of consciousness. It's only the mind that divides it all up, separates it, and judges one thing as good and another as bad. It's the mind's job to make a map of reality, to form beliefs about it. This is an important survival function. Being able to describe our experience helps us understand it and communicate it.

But we make an error when we mistake the map for the territory, when we become so psychologically identified with the mind and its belief structures—which is how the ego is formed—that we fail to see what the anthropologist Gregory Bateson called "the pattern that connects." We miss the forest for the trees. We get so caught up in the description, in the words, that we fail to grasp the significance of what the words are pointing to. We lose the taste, the flavor, of the underlying experience.

The Secret of Dealing with Problems

Inner freedom comes as you let go of your identification with the ego and the beliefs which sustain it, and find your identity instead in the wholeness, the harmony, that is at the heart of existence. It involves a fundamental shift in perception. This shift happens naturally as you get centered and grounded in your body, as you learn to be still, to be sensitive to the creative source, or intelligence, that is behind appearance and manifestation.

You live less and less from your mind, from the sense of a separate ego, or "me," struggling, with all the other egos to find an elusive security in an insecure world. Instead, you begin to live more from an innate knowing, an intuitive sense that you're absolutely okay as you are, that life is inherently good, and that everything is happening as it's meant to be. You begin to live from your heart, your spiritual center, in other words.

Whether you pray, meditate, do psychotherapy, practice yoga, follow the Twelve Steps, live as a Buddhist, Christian, Muslim or Jew, or study the *Course In Miracles*, it doesn't really matter. All of these paths, so long as they are grounded in reality, so long as they help you become more compassionate, more present, have the potential for moving you closer to the freedom and joy that are your birthright.

They help you get to the place where you're no longer so focussed on or obsessed with problems. You're less in your mind, more in your actual, body-based experience of reality. You're quieter and more at peace within. You're more committed to living creatively, to fulfilling your mission in life, your vision, whatever your vision may be.

There is a technique that can help, however, when you're stuck with a problem. This especially applies to a recurring problem, a situation that seems to crop up again and again for you. Try asking yourself, "What is my lesson here?" When the same problem keeps coming up in our lives, it's usually because it's trying to teach us something. There's something we need to learn.

When our most intimate relationships keep causing us strife and grief, for example, there's clearly something we're doing that's contributing to the pain. As I said in the chapter on relationships, it's usually self-will that gets in the way. Because we don't trust that things will work out just fine if we just give the problem some time and space, we tend to contract, to harden, around our own wants and needs. The great lesson in relationship is to let go of our willfulness. It's to soften, to open our hearts.

When you start to probe for the particular lesson that's there for you in any given situation, you'll find—often to your amazement—that many of the problems you've been grappling with simply clear up in the process of life itself. Miracles, big and small, will often happen. Insights and unexpected solutions come. At other times, things that you would have once considered a problem are simply—when you really look at them—no longer an issue.

You begin to understand that the secret to solving problems doesn't lie in having more money, or a different job or relationship. Rather, it's in bringing all your energy, all your creativity and focus, to the moment at hand. As you learn to live each moment with this depth of commitment and presence, the money manifests when it's needed, the relationships have a chance to unfold authentically, organically, and everything you do becomes inherently much more satisfying and rewarding.

Then, as this experience of inner freedom and committed purpose deepens for you, you become more available to help others with their problems. You can serve. More than anything else, it's this ability to really be there for others—especially in ways that help them find their own answers and solutions—that is the sure sign you're doing well on your healing journey.

Be very clear about what you say you want, because the chances are good you'll end up getting it!

Chapter 15
Know What You Want

There's a saying from the Book Of Proverbs in the Old Testament: "Happy is the man that finds wisdom." For the purposes of this chapter I'm tempted to re-phrase that into, "Happy is the man who knows what he wants."

Wisdom, as the Random House dictionary informs us, is having the power to discern or judge what is true or right. To be able to make intelligent, accurate judgments, in turn, presupposes a certain degree of inner clarity. Before you can choose wisely or make a sound judgment, especially around a matter that may significantly affect the course of your life, you must be in touch with your inner needs and values. You must know what you want. You must know what is most important to you.

Psychotherapy and counseling offices all over the nation are filled with people who, when pressed, will say they don't know what they want. They not only don't know, they are confused. They have many conflicting wants and desires, and a variety of considerations—guilt, judgments, doubts—about each of them. This lack of certainty about what we really want may be one of the major reasons for our *angst*, the mental, emotional, and spiritual suffering we experience in our lives.

People who are very clear about what they want may have doubts at times, but as a rule they're not controlled by their doubts. The goals they have for themselves, their vision of what they want for their lives, provide a focus for their energy. Problems and other obstacles tend to be swept aside. The more powerfully clear the goal, or vision, the more attainable it becomes. Ask anybody who has achieved something worthwhile in life, something of value and meaning to them, and they'll tell you that, as the vision became clearer, so the possibility of its attainment loomed larger and larger.

This is why having dreams and setting goals can be so inspiring and energizing. "Imagination is more powerful than knowledge," said Albert Einstein. He was referring to the fact that knowledge tends to be intellectual, dealing in abstract mental concepts, whereas imagination is the ability to form images and pictures, with associated feelings and sensations. Knowledge describes reality in the mind, imagination actually creates it.

The more vivid the imagined picture, the desired state, the more real it seems. You begin to taste it, feel it, smell it, even—almost—hold it in your grasp. When the image of the thing you want is very strong, it's only a matter of time before the vision or dream you've been building and nurturing in your mind begins to manifest itself in reality, proving the truth of Einstein's saying.

Taking the Time for Inner Reflection

People who are very worldly, who aren't given to reflection or contemplation, who have little interest in an inner life, generally don't have the same problem with knowing what they want as do people who are more spiritually-inclined. When we're focussed only on looking outward, what we want usually becomes fairly clear over the process of time: we want physical comfort, material security, success in our career, harmony in our relationships—and, if we're especially ambitious (or insecure!), perhaps even wealth, prestige, and fame.

Sooner or later, most of us discover that to look outwardly only is not enough. No matter how much we may accumulate of the things of the world, so often our inner hunger remains unsatisfied. Money can buy a peaceful environment. It can allow us, if we have enough of it, to jet away to exotic and healing locales, or insulate ourselves from the troubles of the rest of the world. But money can't buy inner peace. Money can buy the best health care available, but it can't buy health itself. It can buy companionship, but it can't buy love. It can buy pleasure, but it can't buy joy. It can buy a good funeral, but it can't keep us from dying.

Money can buy all manner of outer things, but peace, health, love, and joy are all inner experiences, states of being, and there's no way we can manipulate them or make them happen. We can take drugs to get a temporary feeling of peace, of contentment—and even of health—but then the feeling is dependent on the drug. When the drug wears off, so does the experience. Moreover drugs, as we've already seen, all too frequently result in dependency and a host of harmful physical, emotional, and social side-effects.

Crisis as a Wake-Up Call

As we get older, these truths become more evident to us and we tend to become more reflective. Sometimes all it takes is a crisis in our lives, such as the loss of someone we love, or a major reversal in our health or fortunes, and we begin to turn inward.

The crisis serves as a wake-up call and we face, finally, our own insecurity, the fact that, in spite of any material or worldly gains we may have made, we don't really know ourselves. Moreover, the deeper feeling of spiritual well-being that we yearn for still eludes us. We still remain restless and unhappy within.

It's at such times of personal crisis that the spiritual journey often begins. My own journey, which I spoke briefly of in the Introduction, began with just such a crisis. I was twenty-nine years old, knew what I wanted in my life, was ambitious, hard-working, and under a considerable amount of stress. The problem was that I was not even aware I was stressed until, late one night, while studying for some important exams, I began to suddenly experience pains in my chest and difficulty in breathing.

These physical symptoms were accompanied by extreme anxiety, and then panic. I was convinced I was having a heart attack. That night I was afraid to fall asleep for fear that I would die. For many nights thereafter, in fact for almost six months, that fear haunted me. I didn't trust that I would wake up in the morning, so I'd toss and turn fitfully, afraid to relax, to surrender conscious control of my breath, until finally I'd fall asleep through sheer exhaustion.

I dealt with my fear, and the stress behind it, through meditation. I took a course and learned to meditate. I learned how to slow down. Prior to my health crisis, I'd never wanted to sit down and just be quiet, had never wanted to explore the depth, the beauty, the mystery of the moment. All I'd wanted was to actively pursue, chase after, my various goals and ambitions. But the fear of dying if I didn't slow down, if I didn't learn to relax, caused an urgent shift in my priorities. As someone once said, illness is a big stick—it gets our attention. The health crisis I was going through certainly got mine.

In meditation, I began to experience what were for me extraordinary moments of peace and clarity. A new energy, a new understanding, began to enter my life. I realized I'd known such moments of peace and quiet when I was a young boy working on a dairy farm in New Zealand. I'd often go out and sit under the trees on a hillside at the back of the farm. From there I could gaze at the fields laid out before me, and at the mountains in the distance, and just bask in the peace and tranquility of my pastoral environment. But meditation showed me that I could find that same quality of peace anywhere, at any time, so long as I was in a reasonably quiet place.

I'd also begun to read spiritual books and they informed me that it was possible to live with that quality of inner peace. I could have it, or have access to it, on a daily basis, no matter where I was or what I was doing. The writings of people like Krishnamurti, Herman Hesse, Alan Watts, and others all pointed to there being something deeper in life, something mysterious and sacred, and that it was somehow tied in with my real nature, with who I was behind all my ideas about myself.

Through my spiritual inquiry and my meditation I could awaken to my inner Self. I could become more enlightened. I could be a whole and happy human being.

Defining Your Spiritual Goals

It's one thing to want enlightenment, it's another to know what enlightenment actually is. And here, of course, lies the trap, the difficulty, for all of us on a spiritual path. It's relatively easy to define material, or worldly goals. True, when we don't really know ourselves or are at a time of transition in our lives, it can be difficult even to do that. But at least the choices are there, even though we may be uncertain as to which choice we should make.

To try and define a spiritual goal is much more difficult, however. This in part explains why so many people who are on a spiritual path seem lost and confused, caught between two worlds. They neither know what they want in the ordinary, everyday material world, nor are they clear about their spiritual objectives.

It's difficult to define spirituality because you're dealing with something that is, by definition, non-material in nature. Indeed, the first thing that is often said of spiritual experience is that it is "ineffable." It's literally beyond description. We may speak of having a feeling of unity, of joy, of peace, of beauty, of timelessness, yet how do you actually describe these feelings, let alone turn them into goals, objectives, or states of being that you can actively pursue?

The fact is they cannot, in the end, be described or pursued—at least not in a way that you can then take the description and replicate it in order to have the experience yourself. You can tell someone what it feels like to ride a bicycle, and then show them how to do it so they can experience riding a bicycle for themselves. But they still have to get on the bicycle and do it. The fact is that learning to ride a bicycle, for most people, takes only a short time. It is a relatively attainable, easily accomplished, experience.

You can also instruct someone in the mechanics of meditation, but learning the techniques of sitting and being still doesn't necessarily guarantee that they will bring peace or bliss. Some people, especially if they have unresolved psychological or emotional problems, may meditate for years and never experience these deeper states of well-being, let alone discover what it is to have a truly quiet, spacious mind. Rather, their experience tends to be one of restlessness, agitation, of fighting with their mind.

Learning to sit in meditation does pave the way to spiritual insight, however. It's a way of making yourself more receptive to something deeper, to the experience of something new, something that's beyond your direct control. In fact you have to let go of control, you have to surrender your sense of personal self and all the thoughts that reinforce your ego, in order to touch—or be touched by—that larger realm of consciousness, of presence, which is the essence of spiritual experience.

Those who have difficulty with meditation usually need to learn to let go more, to give up trying to attain anything—especially a "quiet" mind! Meditation is above all a process of not-doing. When you've spent your entire lifetime being active and busy, both mentally and physically, to sit down and not do anything is an enormous confrontation to your habitual way of being. Yet, as I've discussed, this willingness to sit down and face yourself, be with yourself, is the heart of meditation.

Getting Honest with Yourself

The first authentic spiritual experience I had was the one I referred to in the Introduction, when I woke up early one summer's morning and found myself in the most profound state of clarity and stillness I'd ever known. The experience was so pure, there was something so timeless, so exquisite about it, that it stirred in me the desire to have it again. In this way my spiritual journey, which had begun several years earlier with the health crisis, took a quantum leap forward.

Yet for many years after I found myself in the situation I described above. I felt caught between two worlds. I wanted this thing called "enlightenment" and yet I was also a family man, a health practitioner, a businessman. I had responsibilities. It seemed that the more energy I gave to my meditation and my pursuit of enlightenment, the more my worldly life fell apart. The more joy I experienced in meditation, the more problems and conflicts I seemed to have with my marriage and my work.

Conversely, when I shifted my focus and gave attention to these more immediate, physical aspects of my life, I found myself getting busier, more involved in worldly things, in activities, projects, and the many obligations of everyday life. Before long I would feel a sense of burn-out. I found myself missing those times of solitude and quiet reflection that nourished me spiritually.

Because of this conflict, this dilemma that I experienced between the demands and challenges of the world and my deep spiritual yearnings, I know I must have often appeared to others as a rather confused, even lost, person. I certainly felt that way myself much of the time!

The healing of this split came about for me as I began to get more honest about what I really wanted. Part of this meant acknowledging that some of my desires had changed. When I had that spiritual awakening that summer's morning, all I then wanted—I thought—was to attain enlightenment and live a spiritually-rich life. If that meant giving up the pursuit of any kind of worldly ambition or success, so be it. (Although I must admit I thought I could somehow hold onto my worldly desires and still reach my spiritual objective. In true American fashion, I wanted my cake and I wanted to eat it too!)

In the end I did give up a lot I'd gained materially. I let go of the security of my business, my home, my friends, and my community in order to make a spiritual journey to Asia. The journey brought me many unanticipated benefits, and much unexpected disillusion.

One of the things that I learned as a result of my travels was that I didn't just want freedom from conflict so that I could enjoy inner peace and happiness—which was how I defined enlightenment at the time. No, I also wanted to make a success of my life in a more traditional, worldly sense. I wanted to be successful as a healer, a writer, a workshop leader. I wanted some of the rewards of middle class living.

(Like many other seekers who have journeyed to the East and been afflicted with dysentery, and the suffering that comes from constant exposure to over-crowded, noisy, and often squalid living conditions, I discovered that it was far healthier—and infinitely more comfortable—being a yogi in California than in India!)

I wanted stability in my life and, insofar as it was possible, some kind of financial security, especially now that I had a family to support. I had to get very honest with myself about this. True, as I found more and more of the inner security that I'd been seeking for so long, I saw that I didn't need the outer security in the same way. I wanted more material comfort and ease, but my well-being didn't depend on it. My sense of identity was no longer so tied to the outer conditions in my life. I was in touch with a deeper truth within me, a current of energy, of joy, that was always there whenever I stopped and listened for it.

From that current I drew my inspiration, my spiritual sustenance.

Trusting Your Own Judgment

One of my most important lessons in self-honesty—in learning to trust my own judgment, and to respect the desires of others—came when I was traveling in Bali. My teacher, moreover, was a young Balinese boy who could not have been more than nine or ten years old. I was taking a walk by the ocean, picking my way among the rocks, stopping occasionally to explore the tide pools, when I saw the boy approach me. He was carrying an ice-chest, and was smiling and waving in my direction. I knew immediately what he wanted. Like many Balinese, young and old, he made a living—or at least earned pocket money—by selling various goods to Western tourists.

Sure enough, he had something to sell me. "You want buy cold drink?" he said cheerfully, as he came up to me.

"What have you got?" I asked him with a smile.

"Whatever you want," he replied, opening the ice-chest. "Look!" He was clearly happy at the prospect of making a sale.

There were colas and carbonated fruit drinks, as well as a few bottles of mineral water.

"I'll take a mineral water," I said.

He told me the price, which I didn't bother to haggle over and then, with an impish grin, said, "You buy me soda?" He pointed to a Sprite.

"Why don't I buy you a mineral water?" I said. "It's better for you."

He frowned. "Mineral water? I don't like."

"That stuff's loaded with sugar," I said, pointing to the Sprite. "It's not good for you." I guess I thought that if I was buying, I had the right to dictate what he should drink. After all, I was a health practitioner, and considered myself quite knowledgeable about nutrition.

But he felt differently, and shook his head. He looked me right in the eye. "Mineral water good for you." He jabbed a small finger at his chest. "Sprite good for *me*."

I laughed. I got the message! I bought him his Sprite, and as he wandered off to his next customer, I sat down to drink my mineral water and reflect on the lesson he'd just given me.

It was a big one. He had made me aware of my own arrogance. So often in the past I'd believed I knew better than others what they should or shouldn't do. No wonder I'd had difficulty knowing my own mind. If I couldn't trust others to know what was good for them, how could I trust myself to know for me?

I don't recollect the boy's name now, but I shall always remember him and the gift he gave me. It would take a few more years yet for that all-knowing arrogance of mine to begin to fade somewhat, but he was the one who initiated the process. I was grateful that by the time my own son was born and became old enough to think and choose for himself, I was more able to honor him.

His mother was the one who taught him to listen to his "inner code," and to trust his own feelings and desires. It wasn't the way I'd been raised, which explains, I think, why I struggled so much with trusting myself when I became an adult. When I was growing up, parents always knew best, even to the extent of what their children should or should not feel.

The Fear of Making a Choice

My own experience has taught me that our circumstances are largely a product of the choices we make in life. Yes, there are many, many people who, because of political or social disadvantages, have only a limited range of choices, of options, available to them. But I could never offer that defense, or excuse. Because I lived in a free society and had received a good education, I had many choices open to me.

What I had to deal with was not the fact that choices weren't available. I had to face my fear of making them.

That meant getting honest with myself about my fear. I was afraid that if I chose the world, if I gave in to my material ambitions, I'd have to sacrifice my spirituality, that connection with the underlying beauty of life that was so essential to my well-being. And I was afraid that if I chose spirituality I would deny myself the things I loved about the world. I was afraid I'd have to say goodbye to the material pursuits and pleasures, as well as my innate sense of excitement and curiosity, that had always made living such a stimulating adventure for me.

What I eventually found was that I couldn't choose one over the other. I couldn't commit myself to one course at the expense of the other. Up until the moment when I saw this, I tended to always be a vacillator, a wobbler. Someone would ask me what I wanted and immediately, if they were at all perceptive, they'd see the hesitation in my eyes, they'd hear the uncertainty in my voice, they'd sense my ambivalence.

In the end I saw that I couldn't help but be committed to my spiritual path, for that was the most important thing to me. And once I made the commitment, embraced it consciously, it didn't, I realize, negate my love for the world. As I've emphasized throughout this book, spirituality that is *embodied* expresses itself—for most of us—in a full and adventurous life that is lived in the world.

In getting more identified with the spiritual reality that is at the heart of life, we find ourselves becoming less attached to outer phenomena, to the flux of events and circumstances. Nevertheless, we're still very much *here*, we're still very much involved in the ongoing challenge of living, learning, relating, and creatively addressing the problems we encounter every day.

Making Spiritual Well-Being Your Priority

The nature of the spiritual journey, then, requires that, sooner or later, you must make some very definite choices. Even though the actual meaning of enlightenment, of freedom, of inner peace, may be unknown or unclear to you (precisely because it is beyond words), you still hold it as a goal.

You still hold to the vision of enlightenment; you still have the dream of a happier, freer life. You must *choose* spiritual well-being, in other words. You must make living authentically—which is to live from your spiritual center—your top priority. It must come before everything else. It must be the center from which everything else in your life radiates.

On the way to the fulfillment of this vision you'll discover that things such as diet, body awareness and exercise, meditation, and learning to be more present in every relationship and situation, facilitates your awakening. You learn that you have to make a commitment to these new ways of being, often at the expense of other habits and behaviors. For instance, you may have to somewhat withdraw yourself from the world, at least for awhile. You may have to give up, or eliminate, some of your worldly attachments and activities so that you have more time and energy for inner work.

Yet as you go further along the path, you'll come more and more often to the place where you see that you no longer have the luxury of choosing. This is yet another paradox. First, you must make a choice, you must choose the spiritual journey. Then as you proceed, you find out that you really don't have a choice! What happens is that as you get more focused in your life, the options before you are not so wide-ranging any more. It becomes clearer and clearer to you that you have a certain mission in life, a certain responsibility. You're here to do a certain thing, and it's time you got on with it.

It's the ego, the small, personal self with all its emotional programming, its hopes, fears, needs, and insecurities, that is continually toying with an endless variety of choices and options. It's the ego that thinks it might be better off leaving this relationship for that, ending this career in order to try something else, moving from this town to a new one—the geographical cure!— and so on.

It's the ego, the small, personal "I," that is constantly choosing one thing over another in its endless search for a more secure identity, in its relentless quest for happiness, for some form of permanent peace and satisfaction.

In the End, There is No Choice

As you heal yourself more deeply, you get freer of the ego and its worries and concerns. Instead, you live more from an inner well-being, a source of wisdom that has its origin beyond the mind, beyond beliefs and ideas, beyond choice. What this means in practical terms is that the choices you need to make in life start to become clearer. You get a glimpse of the truth behind Krishnamurti's famous statement, that, "When you live this way, with this kind of awareness, there is no choice."

As you learn to live out of your real nature, so that you're more consciously and creatively alive in the present, you see what has to be done in any given moment and you simply do it. The example Krishnamurti liked to give had to do with a house on fire. When you suddenly notice that your house is burning, you don't sit around and decide whether you're going to do something about it. No, you jump into instantaneous action. There's no choice. Similarly, when you see a child in danger, you run to help it, you do whatever is necessary. Such immediate, choiceless action is intelligence, it is love in action.

It's one thing to act without choice—or, put another way, to make the only intelligent choice—when faced with a crisis like a house on fire or a child in danger. But what about normal, everyday life, the many mundane situations and problems that require your attention?

After all, most of us are not yet free of our egos, even though we may be getting freer. Daily, we still find ourselves confronted with all kinds of choices. When it comes to knowing what you want, for example, what about that job you have which, while it's not unbearable, is not truly fulfilling either? Or that relationship which, while aspects of it work reasonably well, still lacks something vital, is still not what you know it could be?

In life you'll often be required to compromise, to make trade-offs, to negotiate, to give up something in order to have something else. If you can do this and still feel good within yourself, then it's not a problem. But you should question the compromise or the trade-off you're making if it leaves you feeling resentful, dissatisfied, unfulfilled. Too much compromise, or the wrong kind, will stifle your energy and lead to a mediocre existence—and nothing will kill your spirit and your creativity more than mediocrity.

Getting in Touch with What You Really Want

It's important to be as clear as you can about what you genuinely want for yourself and your life. If you don't know, you should daily ask yourself, "What do I want?" and then, when you think you know, affirm it, say it to yourself over and over again, to see if it's true for you. Remember, the more honest you are about what you want, the clearer you'll get.

As you make these affirmations, your mind will doubtless come up with objections. Some of them may be legitimate, while at other times it may just be your fear—your ego—speaking. The way to distinguish the true voice within you—the voice of your inner Self—is to keep focusing on what you most deeply want, in your heart. If it truly is a heartfelt desire, the doubts and objections put forth by your ego will gradually fall away, and it will become very obvious to you that you're on the right track. You'll feel a sense of rightness, something will "click."

When you're in touch with the truth, you always know it. You feel it in every cell of your body. Whenever you come to an authentic realization, it leaves you feeling clean. You feel a purity, a rightness, throughout your being. When you settle for inauthenticity, however, there's always a residue. You feel unclean, unclear. You know you're not honoring your true Self.

You'll probably find, as I did, that you want many things. It's natural to have wants, to have desires. Desire is an innate human urge, one of our most basic characteristics. Something that stops so many people from having what they really want is the belief that it's "wrong" to want certain things. This seems to be especially common among spiritual seekers. I know that I grew up with the belief that it wasn't okay to ask for what I wanted, that I should be grateful for whatever crumbs of happiness or good fortune chanced to come my way. To ask for more, or to ask for something different, was to be pushy, aggressive and—the worst sin of all—greedy.

Once I saw how much of my spiritual journey was a denial of this unfulfilled aspect of myself—the man who wanted a certain degree of material security, who wanted to do something with his life—it became easier for me to accept the various desires I'd spent so long invalidating and trying to transcend.

The more I embraced them (and this included the petty desires, the selfish ones, the sensual ones), the less of a problem they became for me. The superficial desires, those that turned out not to be important to me after all, fell away once I'd begun to explore them. I began to experience a new sense of freedom. I began to see how much control I had over my life, how much power I had to create the things that really mattered to me.

You'll find this too. As you let go of your judgments and begin to accept your conflicting wants and desires, you'll get closer to the truth of what you really, in your heart of hearts, want. This is what it means to discover your true purpose in life—and the more clear you are about your purpose, the more meaningful your life will be.

Discovering Your Purpose for Being Here

Purpose is a vital word. It refers to the underlying *reason* for which something exists. Discovering our purpose is what we're here for, I believe. Life, by itself, has no purpose. It just is—a ceaseless flow of creation, of endless opportunities and possibilities. It's you who bring purpose and meaning to your life. That is your unique birthright—to discover what you want your life to be, and then to create it in reality.

To know your purpose is empowering because once you embrace it, then choosing what you want becomes relatively easy. You come to the place of no choice, because you'll only want, or want to do, that which serves your purpose. Then you can set goals that are in alignment with your purpose. Purpose is ongoing, it's your reason for being. Your goals, on the other hand, are the short-term objectives, the steps, the means, by which you fulfill your purpose in life.

As we've already discussed, however, the energy of life is non-linear. It's holistic, it moves in cycles. Just as being clear about your purpose leads you to knowing what you want, so knowing what you want leads you more resolutely toward uncovering your true purpose. You move from times of being very clear to times of being not so clear at all, as you uncover your deeper wants and needs. But the overall direction is toward greater clarity and single-mindedness of purpose. This is especially so as you awaken more and more to who you really are, to your own inner authenticity.

It may help you to write down what you want. It can be a very good exercise in getting clear to take a sheet of paper, write down at the top, "What I want..." and then proceed to list, without censorship or condemnation, everything that comes to mind. You should put down even your most off-the-wall or outrageous desires, which includes all the things you've ever felt guilty about wanting.

In addition to writing down your wants and needs, it can be helpful to write down your values. Your values are the things—the ideals, customs, traits, qualities, and behaviors—that are important and meaningful to you. Getting clear about your values helps you discover your purpose, because your purpose—what you're here for, what you want to do with your life—will in some way be related to your values. Your values, in turn, will help you get clearer about what it is you really want.

A third technique, one that can be extremely useful, is to use your power of visualization to paint a mental picture of how your life would look to you if you could have it exactly the way you wished. Sit down, get quiet and centered within, and begin to see it with your mind's eye. This is a more holistic, right-brained approach.

You're literally *seeing* the big picture, sketching a vision of your life as it could be—your ideal scene. Writing down your wants and your values is more linear, more sequential, more left-brained. You're gathering information to help you reach some definite conclusions. With visualization, you simply see the end result. As another of my favorite fortune cookies says, "If you can shape it in your mind, you can find it in your life."

If you're an artist or enjoy graphics, you might actually draw or paint your desired picture, what you want for your life. Or you may prefer to describe it in words, even make up a story about it. Whether you visualize it, paint it, or write it, the main thing is to be clear enough so that you would recognize the scene if it actually manifested in your life. Your ideal scene should be detailed enough that you would know it if you saw it. For some people, this will mean being very detailed and specific. For others, a broad outline, a rough idea, will be sufficient.

So the three methods—listing wants, defining your values, and forming a visual image of your desired reality—complement each other. Each time you work with these three tools you'll notice changes, revisions that you'll want to make. If you work with them over a long period of time—months or years—you'll probably observe continuing changes.

Sometimes, these changes will be more in the nature of refinements, especially once you've begun to get some clarity. At other times, something on the list may change radically, and perhaps even turn into something quite unexpected. This can happen if you've been repressing or denying some deep-seated need or longing which then gets awakened within you.

An Ongoing Process

The process of getting clear about your purpose for being here—and what you need and want along the way to help fulfill your purpose—is an ongoing one. It's a deepening process. It moves in cycles, spirals. Sometimes it will feel as if it's moving erratically, even going in reverse, and yet you'll notice, in your clear moments, that there's a progressiveness to it. There is a direction to it. Your life, you begin to discover, is actually going somewhere. Like a flower coming into bloom, your life is evolving, becoming fuller, riper. It has meaning, and you have a purpose for being here.

It's the allowance for this cyclical pattern, the gradual, organic unfolding of your life, that makes your journey spiritual. To live spiritually means you're in touch with your spirit, your essence, your passion. You're connected to your inner Self, the creative force that gave you life and that inspires every breath you take.

When you have this kind of connection, then goals have meaning. There are many, many books on goal-setting and the art of achieving success in life, but unless your efforts are guided by an inner wisdom you'll never be satisfied with what you achieve in the world. No matter how many goals you attain or how much material success comes your way, there'll still be a longing inside you, an emptiness that no amount of external achievement can fill up.

That inner need starts to be met once you make the choice to heal yourself, to transform your life. That has to be the first and most important thing you want. It's a commitment to living each day with true awareness. As Krishnamurti said once to someone who came to him for counsel: "This has to be your life, sir."

Make your spiritual path your life, make your life your path, and everything else will fall into place.

The Law of Attraction

It won't always be easy and doubts will still crop up, but once you've made the commitment to healing yourself, to becoming fully conscious, you'll attract into your life the people and things you need to help you on your journey. Indeed, once you start making all your choices out of the question, "Does this support my path or not?" you'll be surprised at how magically and synchronistically events will unfold for you.

It's a wonderful thing to know what you want in your life, to have that kind of clarity, that certainty of vision and direction. You come to that clarity, as I pointed out a few pages earlier, by continually asking yourself, "What do I want?" and not censoring your answers. Then, through the human process of trial and error, you'll begin to know what is really in your heart.

As you get clearer, you'll realize that you've always gotten what you wanted. In metaphysics, this is referred to as the Law of Attraction, or the Law of Cause and Effect. It's like water finding its own level. Whatever you're putting out is what you tend to get back. If your basic statement or belief is that you do not want much, or expect much from life, be assured that you probably won't get much. You won't allow yourself to have it, because to allow abundance into your life would be inconsistent with what you believe.

This is why those who resent other people's success continue to feel unsuccessful in their own lives. So long as you resent someone else for what they have or what they are accomplishing, you'll only hold yourself back. This is the mind, the ego, at work. If you resent someone else's financial security for example, believing that they must have "ripped people off" in order to achieve their success, you'll place limits on your own desire for such security. You'll believe that you, too, have to "rip people off" in order to be successful, and you won't allow yourself to do it.

Yet the fact is that the majority of people who are financially successful have arrived at their status through hard, honest work. Deny others their success, and you deny yourself. Allow others to prosper, and you allow yourself to prosper also. It's the same for enlightenment, inner peace, happiness. When you see it in someone else and acknowledge them for it, you give yourself permission to have what they have. But if you refuse to believe that anyone else can be genuinely happy, you're saying, in effect, that happiness is impossible for you, too.

It's also important to differentiate between what you think you want, and what you really, deep down inside, feel or believe you want. You may say, for instance, that you want a good relationship, a partnership with a man or a woman. But if deep inside yourself you have fears around intimacy and entrapment, then it's this core belief that will dictate your experience.

No matter how much you try to have a successful relationship, this inner belief of yours will always tend to get in the way. It will cause you to distance yourself whenever you find that you and the other person are getting too close. You'll tend to become emotionally unavailable, even cold toward the other person, as a way of protecting yourself. In effect, then, you'll actually work at keeping yourself from ever having the kind of fulfilling relationship you say you want.

As you get more honest with yourself and begin to look at those deeper beliefs, fears, and desires that have been running you, then there's less of a split. You become more accepting of your darker, or shadow, side—what psychotherapists call the wounded child within, the disowned self.

You're able to face your own inner pain. This leads to an integration of your energies. You become clearer about what's important to you, what you really want. You feel less of a victim, less like a rudderless ship drifting about aimlessly on the ocean of life. Your life has more of the feel of a true journey, a movement with purpose—the fulfillment of your own unique mission in life.

The Power of Creativity

You'll discover many things as this clarity becomes more real for you. You'll find that you'll be less concerned with material accumulation, with the acquisition of objects for their own sake, and more interested in the creative process itself. When your energy is focussed only on obtaining something, once you have it, then what? Then, unless you know your deeper purpose, you'll simply end up wanting something else in the hope that the new desire, goal, or objective will fulfill you. To live this way is very limited and chronically unsatisfying. The more you get, the emptier you feel.

But when your life is governed by the credo, "I want to create, I want to serve, I want to do something with my life," you find yourself tapping into an infinite source of energy and power. Such a statement is open-ended, limitless in its possibilities. To be creative is to serve, because in the act of creating you're giving back to life. Your creation is your gift to life and to your fellow human beings.

To create is to carry out your purpose in being here. True artists never stop painting just because they have a series of good pictures done, but rather keep on painting because they cannot but do otherwise. To an artist, to paint is to live. Painting is the artist's purpose for being alive. It's how all artists express their sense of spirit, of truth, of the ultimate reality. To rest on their laurels would be to stagnate. It would be to deny the very energy that gives their lives joy and meaning.

You'll find it to be the same in your own life. Knowing what you value, what you want, brings you to clarity of purpose. Your purpose will then seek its natural expression through the creative urge within you. As you allow the creative impulse room to grow and flourish, you'll discover the methods, techniques, and opportunities necessary in order to fulfill your purpose. In this way your life will begin to feel whole. The vision you've had for your life—a vision that you have perhaps held for many, many years—will start to manifest in reality.

It will all begin coming together just as, in your heart, you knew it always could.

Asking the Right Question

This is one of the gifts of growing older. As we age, we generally find ourselves getting clearer about who we are and what's important to us. We feel ourselves getting more focused. It dawns on us that we no longer have forever, and that we'd better get on with whatever it is we're here to do. The discovery that we are, after all, mortal—at least in this body—brings an urgency, a clarity to our lives.

I remember watching a television interview with the San Francisco rock group, the Grateful Dead, a few years ago. The interviewer was asking the group how they had managed to stay together as a top performing band for more than twenty years, and still retain their popularity with their following. "We trimmed the fat," one of them replied. "We got rid of everything that was unnecessary."

Trimming the fat. It's an interesting image, the whole idea of doing away with everything that is unessential in our lives, that gets in the way of our true purpose, our creativity. It's certainly an integral part of the healing journey. We learn detachment, we learn to let go of all that is not us so that our true Self can awaken, so that we can be fully Self-realized.

I've shared a number of tools and techniques for bringing to light your innermost needs and desires. I've emphasized the importance of asking yourself what it is you want most. Too often we are running around looking for "the answer," for what we think or believe we need for our happiness, when we've never clearly defined the question, we've never gotten in touch with our true longing.

According to the Sufis we're each driven by a fundamental question that is the force, the impulse, behind our quest for fulfillment. Discovering what that question is, what it is we are most deeply looking for ("Who am I?" "Am I loved?" "Am I safe?" "Why am I here?" "What do I want?"), orients us, points us in the direction of truth. It leads us to the answer. This is why it's said that the answer is to be found in the question.

It usually takes many years of living in order to come to real clarity. Through a long and often difficult process of trial and error, of pain and suffering, of shattered illusions and broken dreams, you gradually get clearer about what matters to you. You begin to discover what your mission, your purpose is. You find out how you want to serve.

It's an extraordinarily liberating feeling when it starts to come, this sense of purpose. You know it's real, too, when you no longer have to talk about it, when you no longer think about it so much.

Instead, you feel it as something solid within you, solid and yet dynamic, alive. This is the nature of passion, of joy. As I said in the Introduction, it's like a flame burning within you, a bright, steady flame. You take your nourishment, your inspiration from that flame, and you just go about your life and do it; you do what you came here to do.

The results—what you're accomplishing with your life, the people you're helping, the satisfaction you're deriving—speak for themselves.

The greatest joy in life is to be doing what you love.

Chapter 16
Do What You Love

This chapter is related to the previous one, for if there's a secret to knowing what you want, it lies is in discovering what you love. Once you know what you love most in life—and make the commitment to honoring that—then it becomes relatively easy to decide what you want. What you want will always, invariably, be influenced by what you love.

Love and purpose go together. In the previous chapter we saw how, by continually asking yourself what it is you think you want, you get closer to what you really want. As you get clearer about your values, about what's most important to you, so you get more clarity about your purpose in being here, what you want to do with your life.

Another way of approaching this quest for your true purpose is to find out what it is you love most, and then set your life up so that you can do what you love. Some people are fortunate in that they're able to devote pretty well their whole lives to what they love. Their love may be music, art, literature, teaching, health care, social work, farming, parenting—any number of careers or callings. Because of favorable circumstances, or because they're willing to pay the price to make whatever sacrifices may be necessary, they give their lives over to what they love.

Most of us, though, are not born into, nor are granted, the kind of favorable circumstances which allow us to spend all our days doing only what we love. Few of us have, for instance, the kind of financial independence, the freedom from having to earn a living, that allows us to do whatever we might please with our time.

You usually have to trade-off, to some degree. You can live with a trade-off if your most important needs are being met. You might, for example, take a job that falls short of being your ideal career in order to pay your bills. Knowing you have your bills paid then gives you the peace of mind you need for your creative work, for the writing, painting, music, hobby, or craft you really love to do. And you can still hold to the vision of, one day, making the thing you love your full-time work or career.

Compromise, as we saw in the last chapter, only becomes a threat to your well-being when you make concessions that don't serve you, and you end up getting nothing of what you want. Compromise of this nature, where you sell out your own beliefs and principles, can literally destroy your spirit, leading to a life of mediocrity. Thoreau spoke of people living lives of "quiet desperation." Mediocrity is a sure downward spiral into desperation. Don't make the mistake of settling for mediocrity in anything. You'll end up miserable and unhappy. If you're not going to pour all of yourself, your energy and talent, into a project, find something else to do, something that does bring out the highest and best in you.

In many ways, all of life is business. Negotiation and trade-off is the name of the business game. But some things are non-negotiable. Trade your time and your labor, by all means, in order to get the money or whatever else it is you need. But don't trade your soul.

Don't Waste Your Life

Krishnamurti who, in his own unique way, lived a full and vibrantly creative life as a spiritual teacher and philosopher, often spoke out against mediocrity. I once heard him define the word in terms of its ancient Greek roots. It meant, he said, "To climb half-way up the mountain."

The metaphor of climbing only half-way up the mountain is an appropriate one for the spiritual journey, given that the journey is often spoken of as an ascent, a climbing toward a pinnacle of human evolution. You can't reach the top of the mountain by being mediocre, or half-hearted. You must climb with energy, enthusiasm, and a willing spirit. You must be total in your effort and your commitment.

Anything less than a total effort and you'll fall short of your goal. "Don't waste your life," Krishnamurti often counseled people who came to him. To make a practice of only going half-way up the mountain—whatever particular "mountain" you may have chosen to climb, whatever goal you may have set for yourself—is to waste your life. Few things are as tragic as a wasted life.

Often we hesitate to plunge into our lives because we fear we may not succeed. The fear of success, whatever the psychological reasons underlying it, is a big one for many people. Yet there's a beautiful saying in the *Bhagavad Gita*, the holy book of the Hindu people: "It's better to fail at your own *dharma*, your own mission in life, than to succeed at someone else's."

Better, in other words, to not achieve as much as you'd like doing what you love, than to attain material success doing work you don't care about at all. When you're doing what you love, there's a sustaining joy in the work, regardless of whether the outcome of a particular project is "successful" or not. But when your heart's not in the work you're doing because it's not really "you," then, even though you may make money or be considered "successful," you won't be happy. Your soul will suffer.

What the *Bhagavad Gita* is really saying is that, to be happy, you must be yourself. If you think you've got to be like someone else in order to be happy, you're missing the whole point of existence. This is an important teaching to remember, especially given that we live in a society where there's so much media pressure to look, dress, and act a particular way.

Doing What Inspires You

Ramana Maharshi, the Indian sage, was frequently asked by seekers what method of meditation they should adopt, or what spiritual practice they should follow. He often replied to these questions with the statement, "Do what inspires you. That is always the best way."

This is beautiful, simple wisdom. When you feel inspired by something, you're literally filled with spirit, the creative energy of life as it manifests in and through you. It's this quality of spirit you feel and evince that makes you uniquely you. This spirit, or energy, is synonymous with love. You can't feel love, you can't express love, without a corresponding feeling of being inspired from within.

When Ramana said to do what inspires you, he might equally have said, "Do what you truly love." To do what you love is to be uniquely, uncompromisingly yourself. When you're doing what you love to do, an energy moves which brings you into alignment with your true nature, your deepest Self. You naturally find yourself getting quiet, at peace within. All your energies become focused. Your creativity begins to spontaneously express itself. Physical tensions dissolve, and even painful or limiting health conditions often cease to be a problem, at least for the time being.

A wonderful example of the power of inspiration can be seen in the case of Morihei Ueshiba, the founder of *aikido*. When he was in his old age he was so crippled with arthritis that he had to be helped by several younger men onto the mat. Once there, though, he was in his element—where he loved to be—and an energy that was far greater than anything he could muster himself took over, and literally transformed him.

On the mat, Ueshiba embodied the Master—so ageless, so powerful, so invincible that he could defeat as many as ten attackers, all much younger and stronger than he, without seeming to exert any effort at all.

Taking Time for What You Love

One of the things you'll notice about genuinely happy people is that they take time, invariably each day, for doing what they love to do.

Their love may be something as basic as gardening, working with the earth, or they may love working with machines, with things mechanical. Or they may love to write, to paint, to compose, to create. They may love to care for physical environments, to decorate, to keep house. They may love working with people, helping them, encouraging them, relating with them, serving them. They may love solitude and reflection, spending time in nature, taking long, contemplative walks in the woods, or the hills, or by the seashore.

When you're doing what you love, you're naturally in meditation. Your mind becomes quiet without any trouble as your attention gets absorbed by the object of your love. A deeper movement of energy begins to stir. Your heart opens effortlessly as your interest, your creativity, is stimulated. A harmony begins to develop as you feel more and more at one with the moment. and with what you're doing. There's a sense of delight, of anticipation—and, underneath it all, a profound feeling of peace and contentment.

To be engaged in doing what you love is really no different than being in love with another person. There's the same quality, or feeling, of union—of the two, lover and the object of love—becoming one. To find this union within yourself and in your relationship to life is the goal of all spiritual work. Your love relationships actually help you come to this spiritual union, so long as you remember that that's their deeper purpose.

Spiritually, this was always the purpose of marriage. The tradition of marriage was created, long ago, as a sacrament by which men and women, through their union with each other, could come closer to union with God, with their true Selves. This is the meaning of the words, "And the two shall become one."

This also reminds us of why the healing journey is above all a spiritual journey, because in healing we're seeking the resolution of conflict, of duality, of dis-ease. We want the feeling of oneness, or union, in our body, mind, and spirit. When we are sick or in pain we feel pulled, divided, torn. Our body feels one thing, our mind resists it and wants something different, and our spirit has its own yearning.

Love is the healing factor. It's the glue that brings it all together, that unites and bonds the disparate elements. Love heals the split between inner and outer, between the spirit and the flesh. Your love for spirit, for the experience of the infinite, helps free you from the limitations of your body, enabling you to transcend your worldly problems and get some perspective on them. At the same time, your love for the world, for humanity, is what brings you back into your body, into the physical realm—yes, with all its conflict and suffering—where your spiritual insight can express itself in practical and useful ways.

Discovering what it is you love to do and taking time for it each day facilitates this healing. It helps you experience the sense of union, of oneness with Self and creation. A person in love—whether with another human being, or with their vocation, or simply in love with life—is a happy person. When love is present, there'll still be problems and occasional crises to be dealt with, but there's no paralyzing fear, no deep, dividing conflict.

The ego, the individual, separate "self" with all its anxieties and insecurities, is temporarily dissolved into the wholeness, the fullness, that arises when you're established in a larger sense of Being.

Distinguishing between Talents and Gifts

In making the commitment to honoring what it is you love in life, it can help to distinguish between your talents and your gifts. A talent is a natural ability or aptitude for something. Most of us have a number of talents, certain things we tend to be good at, or skilled at doing. You may have a talent, for instance, for cooking, or mechanical work, or putting people at ease in social situations. You may have athletic ability, good eye and hand coordination, which makes games like tennis come easily to you. You may have a talent for art, music, writing.

The talents you have, your aptitudes, are influenced to a large degree by your physical, mental, and emotional make-up. It's unlikely, for example, that a short, squat, and poorly coordinated individual would possess any talent for ballet. By the same token, someone whose mind, whose way of thinking, is more right-brained, who thinks more in terms of the big picture and relies on intuition rather than logical and analytical thought for decision-making, may not make a good draftsman or computer programmer. Both these occupations require a more left-brained, linear approach.

Knowing what your talents are helps you find your place and make your way in the world. It can help ensure you're doing the kind of work that will be right for you, that will go well for you. If you want to take up some new activity or endeavor and you realize you have a talent for it, then you can be more assured of success with your new venture, should you pursue it all the way.

What's interesting about a talent—and makes it quite different from a gift—is that if, for some reason, you don't use it or develop it, it's not necessarily a negative thing. As I indicated, most of us have a number of talents and usually, at some point in our lives, we have to make a choice as to which one—or ones—we're going to cultivate. Few of us have the time to explore every occupation or activity for which we happen to have a talent.

As a personal example, I've always had a natural talent, or flair, for drawing. At one time I explored it more fully by beginning a course in drawing. But soon after I found out that I had the potential to draw well, I made the conscious choice not to go any further with it. I realized there were other things I wanted to do more. I had other goals and priorities. I knew that if I went through the rest of my life and never took up a sketch pad again, it would be okay. And yet I also knew that there might come a day when I would take up drawing again.

This brings me to the discussion of what a gift is, because a gift is something very different from a talent. As I indicated, a talent is something you have largely as a result of your physical, mental, and emotional make-up. In this sense it's material in nature, very physical. It's shaped by conditions and circumstances. A talent means you have an aptitude for something, but it doesn't necessarily mean you have a gift for it. When you exercise a talent, you may become competent, even excellent, but you won't necessarily shine.

There are many talented singers, for example—individuals who have the equipment, who possess a good voice—but few gifted ones. There are many fit, talented athletes, but few who astonish us with their natural ability to excel. There are many talented poets, but few who move us deeply and profoundly. There are talented statesmen, politicians, world leaders, but few who, through their words and their actions, inspire us with any kind of deep love or admiration.

A gift is not a physical aptitude, but is something that comes from another realm altogether. It's a unique quality or attribute *given* to you by spirit, by life, by the intelligence that created you.

To find out what you're gifted in, what gift you have to bring to the world, may be one of the most healing discoveries you'll ever make. To do what you're gifted at is to fulfill your inner spiritual urge to create. It's a sharing of the bounty that's within you. When you give your gift to others in this way, you spread joy wherever you go. Then there's no doubt about the meaning or purpose of your life.

Following Your Bliss

Everyone has a gift of some kind, something unique that has been given them. If you don't yet know what your gift is, then don't despair. As you go further on your spiritual journey, you'll get more in touch with what's inside you, with why you're here. Your gift may be something that will affect, and possibly even change, the lives of many, many people, or it may express itself in a much more modest way. If nothing else, your gift may simply be to live your life with integrity, wisdom, and love.

For a gift is above all an expression of love. It's to be inspired, to be moved by spirit. To express your gift is to do what you love. To find out what you love to do and to make the commitment to doing it, is a sure path to joy and fulfillment. Discipline and effort come relatively easily when you feel inspired by something. This is why Joseph Campbell encouraged people to "follow their bliss." On the other hand, if you put energy into doing something that you have no real love for, then the work will feel arduous, and all your efforts will likely come to nought. You may accomplish some material objective, but you won't feel nourished at the level of your soul.

This is how you know whether you're on the right path or not. This is how you differentiate between a talent and a gift. This is how you discover what you love. It's the quality of the *feeling* that is the key. Love is something you feel. You feel it as a quickening, an opening, an expansion of your being. You feel it as a warmth, a fullness, a richness inside you. You feel it, intuitively, as a sense of *rightness*. It may not make sense logically, but something deeper, something that's beyond the rational mind, tells you that what you're feeling is true, and that it's right.

I remember when I was younger it was always difficult for me to make important decisions. I'd seek counsel from others whom I thought could advise me, after which I'd make up a list of all the "pros" and "cons" pertaining to the particular decision I was facing. By the time I got to the end of my list, I had usually reached a logical conclusion. The course of action that made the most sense from a rational perspective would stand out. But—and here's the catch—I always seemed to end up doing the opposite of what logic told me to do!

Why? Because all my logical calculations didn't take into account the feeling element, the emotional factors, the spiritual needs and considerations. My head, in other words (which is where I tended to live), failed to listen to my heart. Becoming aware of this process, of how my heart eventually always won out over my head, made it a little easier for me when I came to future crossroads, to new decision points.

I eventually stopped making up lists of pros and cons, and just began to listen to my heart, my intuition, right from the outset. It eliminated a lot of mental conflict and time-wasting vacillation. If it felt right to do a particular thing—felt deeply right, that is, so that there was a sense of alignment and integrity within me—then I did it. If it didn't feel right, then I refrained from taking action. I waited until I got a clearer sense of inner guidance.

Love Always Knows What to Do

To do what you love, then, is to listen to your inner Self, to what most deeply inspires you. It's to follow your heart. You can ask yourself the question, "What is it that I love most?" and then listen carefully for the answer. Feel for the answer. To ask yourself what it is that you love is a question that usually doesn't require a lot of repetition. Love is inborn, innate. Most of us know what we love, if we'd be but honest enough with ourselves to face the truth.

Knowing what you want is something different. Most of your desires spring from the mind, from your ideas and beliefs about what will make you happy. These ideas and beliefs are often erroneous, or at the very least misguided, as proven by the fact that the happiness derived from them tends to be short-lived. But to know what you really love—as opposed to what you want, or desire—is to get in touch with an energy, a movement of spirit, that's already there, within you.

Again, on a personal note, I've always loved to express my creativity through writing, especially through writing prose like this, words that are meant to stimulate, inspire, and guide others to be more of who they really are. Give me a desk in a quiet room with a window that looks out on some hills, some trees and the sky, and I'm a happy man. I've known this about myself for many, many years. Each time I sit down to write, though it may be difficult starting at times, and though some days don't go as well in terms of productivity, the knowledge that I'm doing something I love is always there. Each time, the feeling is always fresh and new, and yet it has a timeless quality to it too, for that's the nature of love.

I also love to just sit and be, to meditate, to commune with spirit, with the beauty and the fullness of the moment. These are the times when I feel most at peace, most content within myself. In these moments I am in touch with creation, the source, with eternal *Being*. When I'm connected to the source like this, my true Self, I feel deeply and profoundly loved within.

At such times I am renewed and made whole. I discover again, that I'm loved by life, by that which has created me, and that no harm can befall me, no matter what may seem to be happening in my life or circumstances. Out of this sense of renewal comes inspiration, the desire to move out into the world again, to express the love that I feel inwardly through writing, healing, and relating to others. These are some of the ways that I share my love.

"Seek ye first the Kingdom of God," Jesus taught, "and all these things will be added unto you." You, too, will begin to experience a healing as you allow yourself to be moved by the energy of love—which is spirit's Kingdom—within you. Because of the tendency of the mind to attract to it what it thinks about, if you know what you want, you're virtually assured of getting it. If, at the same time, what you want is inspired by love, by a feeling of warmth and beauty deep in your heart and soul, then you can be assured of happiness and fulfillment.

Love is the very nature of happiness and fulfillment. These two qualities don't lie in objects, in obtaining or acquiring things. They are the essence of love itself. When you listen and feel for what you love, for what is true inside you, for what it is that really moves you, then the very act of listening and feeling is itself love.

Then, once you're in touch with the feeling, you'll soon enough discover what to do with it. Love always finds a way to express itself. It can't do otherwise.

Taking care of your physical environment and your personal and business affairs creates stability in your life, making it easier to stay connected to spirit, to your higher Self.

Chapter 17
Take Care of Business

Once you've begun to accept that the healing journey you're on is a spiritual one, it changes your relationship with life. You begin to live with a different perspective. As the change deepens, it becomes more of a genuine transformation. You're no longer the person you used to be—a prisoner of your childhood emotional programming, social conditioning, and the various beliefs with which you grew up.

Instead, you start to become the person you *really* are, beneath all that conditioning. Your spirit, your authentic Self shines through and expresses itself in a way that is uniquely yours. This is what it means to fulfill, or actualize, your own innate potential. This is the "cure" that every suffering human being seeks.

What becomes most obvious with this transformation is that you are no longer so identified with what's happening outside you, in the everyday world. You are no longer such a helpless player in the drama of living—the drama that was once perhaps so consuming for you. You've discovered that there's a reality beyond what your ordinary eyes see, and you live more from that reality. You're still very much in the world, but you're no longer *of* it to the same degree. Worldly conditions and circumstances no longer have the same seductive hold over you. Your identity, your sense of well-being and security, come from a deeper spiritual source.

Throughout this book I've emphasized how spiritual well-being is the key to a truly happy, creative life. I have shared, too, how my own experience has helped me see how important it is to bring our spiritual insight into the everyday world of home, work, and relationships. As Jean Klein says, "You may be able to play Hamlet in your kitchen, but can you play him on the stage?" Or, in a more popular expression, can you walk your talk? In this chapter I want to explore more fully how daily life itself contributes to healing and awakening.

Bringing Your Enlightenment into Daily Life

Ram Dass, the popular American spiritual teacher who did so much to inspire the searching generation of the Sixties, and whose work of compassionate service to others continues to this day, often makes the point, "Come on gang, it's time to come down off your meditation bench and learn your zip code." This is his way of pointing to the wisdom of attending to the needs of everyday life. When we open to the unitive state, the transcendent reality we call "God" or "spirit," it's all too tempting to want to remain there. When we have tasted the bliss of Divine presence, the temptation to escape the world with its endless round of challenges and responsibilities is often strong indeed.

Listen to these words from Karlfried Graf Durckheim in his book, *Zen and Us*. "A day inevitably comes when we realize that the peace we seem to have found outside life's contradictions is actually the peace of indolence. Repressing our true nature was one way of failing to become a complete human being—and we fail again now if we try to pretend that we have no ego, that we are not in the world... We are forced again and again to face up to the ego and our human destiny."

He goes on to say, "It's true (with awakening), that the objective world has become 'transparent' once and for all, allowing Being to show through—but the real task now is to bring Being into everything we see and do, to make existence fully real in terms of Being. It's this new sense of responsibility toward a new world, and not merely the breaking of the old one's spell, that makes the Zen experience satori."

Satori is the flash of enlightenment, the intuitive realization that your real nature is Buddha, or wholeness, and that to be happy, to be at peace, you need only rest in your true nature. Yet your ordinary humanity demands that you be present not only with the unitive state, the truth of your inner Being, but also with the multiplicity of life, the diversity of everyday experience.

Zen speaks of this as, "chopping wood and carrying water." To chop wood and carry water is to go about the normal business of living. It's to bring your enlightenment into the marketplace. It's to be an ordinary person, doing the kinds of things that ordinary people do to make a living, to provide for their well-being and physical security, to educate themselves, and to enjoy whatever recreational pursuits they may choose to follow. The more enlightened, or conscious, a person is, the more care and sensitivity they bring to their daily tasks and responsibilities.

In this way the world is healed. You start out as an ordinary, unawakened person, and then one day, for whatever reason—due to a crisis, due to the influence of another awakened individual, due to your own inner urge for freedom finally expressing itself—you wake up. You start to become attuned to the Reality, the immensity, that underlies all appearances. And the more awake you become, the more you see the need for bringing your wakefulness into your everyday affairs. This, you realize, is what true spirituality is about. This is what it means to live your understanding

The understanding I'm talking about is not intellectual understanding. Indeed, you begin to grasp that the more you *think* you know, the less you really know. You see that when you let go of all you think you know, then and only then, do you know something. And what you know, as we've seen, is really quite beyond words.

It's this kind of intuitive understanding of the nature of reality that leads naturally to humility and a simpler, saner way of living. Even though you're now awake, where before you were once quite asleep, you're still perceived—by the eyes of the world—as very much an ordinary person. Indeed, ordinariness, you discover, is what you were seeking all along. (And you thought you wanted to be someone special!) It's a wonderful freedom to have nothing to prove, nothing to boast about. It's quite a paradox at first. Here you are, not trying to convince anyone of anything and yet people, for some reason, find you more convincing than ever. How extraordinary!

Becoming ordinary again gives you an appreciation for the meaning of the well-known Zen saying, "Before enlightenment, mountains are mountains and rivers are rivers. During the process of waking up, mountains no longer seem to be mountains and rivers no longer seem to be rivers. But after enlightenment, mountains are once again mountains, and rivers are once again rivers."

It's also said in Zen that, after enlightenment, nothing changes and yet everything is somehow different. What is different, of course, is the clarity and freedom you experience as a natural by-product of being awake, and the joy and compassion toward others that begins to flow out of this freedom.

What is different is that before, you always felt a little empty, a little hungry. You always felt that something was missing in your experience, that something was eluding your grasp. You continually looked outside yourself for that something, trying to find it in relationships, in work, in money, in things, in activities, in causes. Still, that vague emptiness that the American writer and Zen teacher, Peter Mathiesson, called "the hollow at the end of every breath," remained.

Once spirit, or Being, has become a reality for you, then even though you may forget it at times, even though you may get distracted, you realize at some level that it's always here. You just have to stop and be still, and open yourself to it and you soon feel its healing presence again. It's an actual reality for you, a current of fullness, of substance—not merely an idea, or a vague longing.

The Value of Self-Discipline

Just as when you feel this sense of presence, of harmony, you see the need for going about your worldly activities more consciously and carefully, so getting your daily affairs in order and being more organized in your life helps you be more attuned to spirit.

This is how the split that is so often felt on a spiritual path, the conflict between the spiritual and the worldly life, is healed. The healing comes as you give attention to the practical realities, the conditions and circumstances, of your life. You see this philosophy at work in the wisdom of Jesus' saying, "Render unto Caesar that which is Caesar's, and unto God that which is God's." Keep your checkbook balanced, pay your taxes and bills on time (or as soon as you can!), keep your appointments and agreements with others—and always, always remember who you are. Keep coming back to the source, to spirit, to that underlying sense of presence.

There's a reason why monasteries and ashrams have a daily schedule, or regimen, and why monks and novitiates lead such disciplined, ordered lives. Having everything run in as smooth and orderly a fashion as possible prevents wasted energy. It means you don't have to expend energy in dealing with situations that have been neglected and gotten way out of hand, or in doing the same job twice (or many times over, for that matter).

In your own, more worldly life, you can learn something from the monastic regimen. The more organized you are—without being neurotic, compulsive or obsessive about it!—the more energy you'll have available for enjoying the moment, for doing inner work, or for pursuing an activity or project which really interests you.

The word "discipline" derives from a Latin root which means, literally, "to grasp." It's discipline that enables you to grasp, to learn, to understand something, so that it becomes your own. You can see this meaning in the word *disciple*. A disciple is one who is a student, who follows another, a teacher, in order to learn something—to "grasp" the truth of something. Out of this we get the concept of *self-discipline*. To be self-disciplined is to voluntarily adopt the actions and behaviors that best allow you to learn something you want to know, something that will, in some way, improve your understanding of life and your ability to make your way successfully in the world.

So often we give the word discipline a negative connotation. It implies being forced to do something you really don't want to do, or being bound by uncomfortable and unappealing restrictions and constraints. Of course, if the restrictions are being imposed on you by someone else, then it's natural to have a resistance to them—especially if you've already learned to value and trust your own individuality, your own creative freedom.

When you don't yet know yourself, however, and are still seeking psychological security outside yourself—in beliefs and concepts, or in organizations or relationships—living according to another's rules can have a certain amount of appeal. I joined the New Zealand army at age eighteen and, after six months as an enlisted man, went to officer training school. I loved the order, the ceremony, the discipline of military life. The part of me that was stiff and controlled, that needed to belong to something bigger than myself in order to feel secure inside, found a perfect niche in the army.

I thrived on military life, and the discipline came easily to me. As a young second lieutenant and, later, a captain, I felt important, I felt that I was somebody—and, of course, in the eyes of many of those junior to me (at least the young, naive recruits, if not the weathered N.C.O.s!), I was. I enjoyed giving salutes, and I especially enjoyed receiving them. Being saluted, and being called "Sir," validated my rather inflated sense of myself!

But a year after graduating from officers' school I went to Vietnam, where I served with an artillery unit, first as a gun section commander, and then as a forward observer with the infantry. I was in Vietnam during the Tet offensive of 1968 and my experience there began the disillusioning process for me. For the first time in my life I saw death, and faced the possibility that I could very well get killed myself. It was a rude initiation into manhood. I discovered that the army was not just about brass bands and parades after all, but that its true purpose was much deadlier.

A few years after my tour of duty in Vietnam was over, I left the army. Even though I didn't consciously realize it at the time, my search for my real Self had already begun. But I never regretted my army years, mainly because of all that I learned about myself and my capabilities. The training at officers' school had been demanding and had imbued me with certain standards—relating to physical prowess, dress, bearing, personal organization, and self-discipline—that, in spite of a natural slacking off, have never entirely deserted me.

In fact, I found those same qualities a distinct asset when, many years later, I began to actively explore yoga, Zen, and meditation. It was easy for me to get up early in the morning and sit on my meditation cushion for twenty or thirty minutes, or take an hour to do a series of yoga postures in the late afternoon. Even before the army I'd had a natural tendency to self-discipline. I think it came out of my inborn desire to learn whatever it was I needed to know to make it in the world. The army just gave me more of a form for what it meant to live a disciplined, regimented life. Because of the rules and my desire to get ahead, to be approved of by my superiors, I had lots of practice at the art of being self-disciplined.

In subsequent years, especially when I started some psychotherapy and began encountering some of my shadow self, the feelings and emotions connected with my inner pain, I saw how much of the "discipline" I'd acquired was a defense. I began to see how deeply insecure I was, and how I hid my insecurity behind a solid wall of control and self-discipline. As the wall began to come down, my understanding of what discipline really was began to change. I saw it more as a natural aspect of my inner desire to learn and to grow.

Self-discipline helped me arrange my life in such a way that I could get the most benefit from any new experience I had. The difference now was that there was more balance within me, more fluidity. I could use the control that I'd developed to facilitate my ability to be present, to be attentive to the learning at hand, and I could at the same time relax it so as to allow something new—something that might even have been a little threatening—to enter my awareness.

You, too, will come to the realization, if you haven't already done so, of how important self-discipline is on your own healing journey. John Bradshaw defines self-discipline as "delaying gratification." Through self-discipline you're agreeing to put off something that will give you a temporary feeling of pleasure in order to obtain something else, something that will, eventually, contribute to a deeper and more lasting well-being.

I like Bradshaw's definition because it supports one of the key themes I've been stating throughout this book: as our deeper well-being becomes more important to us, it becomes easier to make the changes necessary to support our healing and transformation.

It's very often the stiffness and soreness we feel in our aging bodies that causes us to finally take up a regular, more disciplined program of exercise. It's our desire to feel good on a consistent basis—to be mentally clear, to feel emotionally stable—that drives us to do something about our addictions and our diet. And it's our longing for the experience of unity, of wholeness—not just while meditating or praying, but throughout our day—that prompts us to work at getting our business and personal affairs in order.

Creating a Daily Routine that Keeps You Centered

Here's a laundry list of suggestions and ideas which, if you put even some of them into practice, will free up your time and energy and help you be more on top of things in your life. It's really my own list that I'm sharing with you. I don't always follow it to the letter because for me, too, it's only a general guideline. I never did like being too tied down, even by my own routine. Yet my routine, such as it is, brings order and stability into my life. It helps keep me centered, and allows me to do things like write books, maintain an active healing practice, teach seminars, be a Dad to my son, and give time to my other relationships, without getting too distracted or harassed.

So, to begin with, rise early—unless to do so is total anathema to you! Rising early gives you a head start on the day—and makes you really appreciate the mornings when you decide to sleep in. Besides, the early morning is the best time to meditate. Everything is quiet at that hour. Once you're awake and your head is clear (nothing like a good cup of tea or coffee to do that!), the presence of spirit can be more readily felt. For many people the morning is also the best time to do creative work, precisely because it's so easy to be connected to spiritual inspiration. When you're in touch with the source, creativity happens naturally.

Do your stretching exercises in the morning if your schedule permits. Otherwise, find time later in the day. What's important is that you do them. Then do something aerobic, like walking, jogging, biking, etc. As I've said, I like to go for a run of two to three miles, an average of four to five times a week.

Eat a good breakfast, along the dietary lines discussed in Chapter Five. Be conscious with your other meals, with lunch and dinner, and any snacks you may have in between. Always remember that your goal with food is to eat for optimal health and energy, rather than for emotional reasons. At night, especially, eat lightly.

Keep your living space clean and organized. Make it a healing environment through the use of light, color, flowers, plants, pictures, and whatever other beautiful things may appeal to you. Beauty, whether in the form of art or nature, points us back to the ultimate reality. Beauty comes from God, and it orients us back to God. The wholeness or perfection we see in someone or something beautiful is but a reflection of the beauty within us. It's the Self seeing the Self. This is why a healing and aesthetically-pleasing environment is so spiritually-renewing.

At your job, no matter what kind of work you do—whether at an office, on a construction site, driving on the freeway, or at home—do it conscientiously. Be as present as you can be at your work. Remember the Zen master's advice, "When washing the dishes, simply wash the dishes." This means keeping your attention in the present. It's unrealistic to expect to stay in the present constantly, but you can be aware when your attention wanders. That awareness brings you back to the here-and-now.

Work, even of the most humble kind, can be a wonderful meditation. The goal of work, from a spiritual perspective, is to learn to do the work without being attached to the fruits of your actions. Learning to be more and more grounded in spirit, in your true nature, while you work helps you do this. It's a matter of remembering the presence of God within you, and then bringing the feeling of that presence into your work, into whatever activity you may be engaged in.

When you're able to do this, work becomes true service, a gift both to you and to those who are benefiting from your labor. Being attuned in this way happens in moments at first, and then more frequently and more consistently as your commitment to your own healing grows. It's your commitment that reminds you to stay connected with what is real, with what is actually so in your life, and not get lost in or distracted by appearances, or by your judgments, beliefs, and opinions about things.

Work as a Spiritual Exercise

I'd like to share a few paragraphs here, again from Karlfried Graf Durckheim. They speak eloquently and succinctly both of the role of work as spiritual exercise, and of what it means to be committed to the spiritual journey. They come from a book of conversations with Durckheim, called *Dialogue On The Path Of Initiation*, by Alphonse Goettmann (Globe Press Books, 1991).

"We only see something when we look for it, and we only find something when we are searching. At all times, in every circumstance, we can develop our inner consciousness, awaken the taste of the numinous. An action as simple as walking can be an excellent medium for learning openness to Being; nothing but conscious walking… It's a matter of feeling the act, not to think about it, but to do it in full consciousness, with the attention directed toward our depth. That is why, among our automatic movements, breathing is such a privileged area. As soon as you follow it consciously, without interference, you can be seized by the divine breath.

"This can be applied to any job. For instance, an accountant who adds numbers all day long. His way of being there while writing those numbers can be a prayer. The fact that his consciousness is occupied by some work does not in any way inhibit contact with Being. The issue is always to know how this particular work that I am doing allows me to train myself in the right attitude to witness to the divine. Look at a bricklayer; the way in which he throws cement on the wall. What a magnificent movement, it's like a dance. For the master mason, there can be a numinous experience in the repetition of this gesture.

"Or painters who make the same movement. I know several for whom it's a true spiritual exercise. The farmer, when he uses his hoe, can make of it a religious act. Look at his face. And the craftsman: the shoemaker, the metalworker. In the workshops where they have worked for ten or twenty years, where they always make the same movements, there is a numinous quality in the atmosphere that opens up your senses as soon as you come in contact with it."

Durckheim goes on to say, a little later, "The problem of attention is nevertheless more difficult during the day; it does not just happen by itself. Permanent vigilance is the fruit of a definitive decision of the individual. It presupposes a decision that comes from the core of your Being as it progresses on the way. The depth of the decision is the only assurance of loyalty to the path that you want to take. It's only when you've truly decided to climb to the summit of a mountain that you'll not turn back at the first sign of fatigue. The depth of commitment is the best assurance of attention."

Entering the Fray

A number of years ago I was staying with friends, John and Letitia Allan, who live near Cambria, on the coast below the Big Sur area of California.

Our conversations always centered around spirit, around what for us was the deepest joy in living. At this time in my life I was still struggling with the split I felt between my spiritual yearnings and my life and work in the world. I wanted to integrate the two more successfully. I still had a tendency to want to escape what I perceived to be the drudgery of ordinary life through seeking out the joy of solitude, of meditative bliss, and I knew that wasn't working for me any more. My challenge, which I've alluded to throughout these pages, was to learn to *embody* my spirituality.

One morning I left John and Tish to go and visit the township of Cambria. While in town I chanced upon a small shop which specialized in selling things Scottish—kilts, tartans, clan mugs and plaques, music tapes, books, and so on. My ancestry is Scottish, from the Orkney Islands, and on an impulse I stopped and went into the store.

A woman was asking the lady behind the counter about her clan, and I realized I didn't know what clan my family belonged to. I asked for a book on clan history so that I could check it out. I felt rather excited as I leafed through the index, looking for our family name. I'd never been too concerned about my roots before, but now it became of great interest to me.

Our name was there, with the spelling only slightly altered (the "a" was taken out, so that it was *Drever*), and we belonged to the clan Sinclair. I found the page on the Sinclairs. They had been in possession of the earldom of Orkney since the late fourteenth century. I looked at the tartan and the crest, which showed a cockerel, and then, to my amazement and my delight, I read the clan motto: "*Commit thy work to God.*"

I felt like it was a confirmation that I was on the right path after all. And whether many of the Sinclairs and their clan colleagues had been genuinely spiritual people or not, at least the influence had been there. I came from, and was heir to, a truly spiritual lineage. I got quite a boost from knowing that. It said to me that I was moving in the right direction in my life. I was, in some small way, fulfilling the destiny my forbears had intended for me. I was honoring the tradition of my clan.

Then, some time later, I had a powerful dream in which the meaning of my destiny—and the challenge of accepting it—became very clear to me. The dream came at a point in my life when I was struggling with bringing my teaching work into the world, while at the same time I was trying to deal with the demands of my practice, the debts I'd incurred, and a host of other demands being made upon me. The stress I was feeling because of all this had caused a flare-up of an old somatic disorder—a queasy stomach and an irritable bowel.

In the dream, I was with my clan, back in a time that was several hundred years ago. We were about to engage another clan, an ancient enemy, in battle. The Chieftain, who was an older man with long, white hair, and piercing yet kind blue eyes, gave me a searching look.

"We're abo't to enter the fray," he said, holding his sword at the ready. "Hae ye the stomach for it, Jimmy?"

I pulled myself up to my full height, and returned his gaze. I gripped my own sword tightly. "Aye," I replied, aware of the gnawing fear in my gut. "My stomach hurts sometimes, but I hae."

I awoke from the dream feeling a sense of my own power, my power to take action, to fight the good fight. The message of the dream was clear. It takes courage to make one's way in the world, to fight for what one believes in. But if one is to live authentically, there's no other choice but to honor one's fear, and summon up the courage. Or, as has been said by others, to feel the fear and do it anyway.

Money

Related to the whole issue of work, and one of the main reasons why most of us go to work in the first place, is money. Money is our chief medium of exchange, and it's one of the ways in which we measure the value of things. With money we obtain the goods and services we need—or desire—for our survival and our well-being. None of us gets very far in the material world—in Caesar's world—without it.

For some reason, it's common for people on a spiritual path to have issues around money. This may be because money is such an emotionally-charged matter for so many of us anyway. Many religious teachings tend to support the notion that spiritual enlightenment and material wealth are incompatible. In many Eastern traditions there's a strong emphasis on the value of renunciation, asceticism, and poverty. From our own Bible come such teachings as "The love of money is the root of all evil," "It's easier for a camel to pass through the eye of a needle than a rich man to get to heaven," and "Blessed are the poor in spirit, for they shall inherit the earth."

Again, speaking of my own experience, I've certainly had my challenges around money. Learning to ask for it in exchange for my services without feeling guilty was a problem when I was new in business. I had the belief that somehow what I was giving people wasn't worth very much—which, of course, came directly out of the doubts I had about my own self-worth.

I didn't manage my money as well as I could have, either. I spent too much, and didn't save enough. I lived day-to-day with no plan or goal for the future, pretty much as an alcoholic or drug-addict lives from day to day, waiting for the next "fix." I'd wait for the next infusion of cash to pay the past due bills—and, if I was ahead of the game, if I had excess funds in the bank, I'd sit back and coast, thinking that everything was okay.

It took me a while to wake up to the fact that I was in denial around money, that financially I hadn't been very responsible. I got used to making money as a chiropractor, and I just assumed I'd always have plenty of money. I didn't stop to think about such things as the costs of divorce and child support, or that the economy might be affected by a recession, and that the health-care industry itself would go through major changes.

My reluctance to come to terms with money in a mature, business-like fashion—which includes planning for the long-term—meant that it continued to be a problem for me. I clung to the belief that the money problems would work themselves out, that they would take care of themselves somehow, provided I remained spiritually-centered within myself. As one of my more practical and grounded friends said, "You rely too much on magical thinking when it comes to money."

What I found was that no matter how often I sat down and felt a wonderful sense of peace in my meditation, no matter how many illuminating insights I had, or marvelous spiritual retreats I went to, the problems of unpaid bills, back taxes, and insufficient funds for the future still remained. They needed to be dealt with. I needed to get more involved in my own business affairs. I needed to take some personal responsibility for them. My money problems were not going to somehow miraculously sort themselves out. I needed to do something. I needed to plan, and I needed to take action.

This is why it's so important to take care of business, to get your everyday life organized and under control, so that it doesn't interfere with or distract from your inner well-being. It's a very fine line, a balancing act at times. It's true that the more established you are in your real nature, in spirit, the less affected you are by the ups and downs of circumstances. As you grow spiritually, the health of your bank account has less and less to do with how you feel about yourself. But until you come to that place where the external conditions of your life no longer exert such a powerful emotional hold on you, it makes sense—pays, you might say!—to be practical and responsible with your money and your business affairs.

You might even call it the Zen of money management. By definition, to live in an enlightened way is to be conscious with everything you do, and that includes the way you handle your money. Money, remember, is a medium of exchange. Exchange means something given in return for something else. In the case of money, it's goods or services that are being provided in exchange for dollars. So long as you're focusing on rendering a service, the money you receive will not only be well-earned, it will also be well-deserved and entirely appropriate.

Once you begin to grasp this attitude of exchange and service, then you'll have more insight into the relationship between spirituality and money. You'll see that it's the *love* of money that is the root of evil, not money itself. It's the inordinate *attachment* to it, at the expense of other, more human and compassionate considerations, that creates misery and suffering.

The reason why the rich man cannot get to heaven is because his attention is focused outside himself, on his hoarded wealth, and not inside, where his natural treasure, the jewel of his own spirit, resides. Due to his continual counting of his assets, his heart is closed to the true beauty in life, the riches that are always here in each moment.

Similarly, it's the poor in *spirit* who shall inherit the earth, which doesn't mean that you need to live in poverty in order to find God. To be poor in spirit is to be open spiritually, free of any conditioned dogmas or beliefs about what is or is not spiritual. It's to have an open mind and heart so that something new can come in. To be poor in spirit is to have the "beginner's mind" that characterizes the Zen approach to life.

Our grandparents (and, for some reading this, our parents), who grew up before the days of easy credit, knew how to deal most effectively with the energy of money. After the cash-rich years of the "Greedy Eighties," we entered the era that has become known as the "Frugal Nineties." We're all having to tighten our belts, and many of the simple, common-sense rules that governed the financial lives of our parents and grandparents have come back into vogue.

This wisdom has to do with learning to enjoy a much simpler lifestyle, finding pleasure in friends and family, and in activities—like hiking, swimming, gardening, tinkering, finding ways to express ourselves creatively—that cost very little. It means focusing on ways to save money, instead of spending it. (One of my great insights was that we don't accumulate cash by spending it!). It means not incurring new debt, and working a little harder to reduce the debt we already have. Above all, it means changing our perspective, putting the physical, emotional, social, and spiritual quality of our life before anything else, especially the material *quantity* that we once thought was going to make us so happy.

After all, from a spiritual perspective, the main reason for seeking financial stability is that it frees up our creative energy, allowing us to get on with our real work in life. It's letting money be the by-product of what we do. It may well be a means to certain ends, but to make money the end itself is a prescription for unhappiness.

Teaching Your Children

Another reason for wanting financial stability is to provide for the welfare and education of our children. If you have children, then you have a responsibility to them. They need to be taken care of on many different levels, especially when they're young.

How children feel about themselves psychologically and emotionally, how eagerly they embrace life and deal with the adventure of living, how sensitive and aware they are in their relationships with others, depends to a large degree on how their parents handle these matters. Whether a child grows up with a spiritual perspective on life or not is also largely due to the parent.

I remember that my parents were not particularly spiritual in any sense, but my mother spoke to me about God when I was very young. She let me know that God was real, and she taught me how to pray. I shall always be grateful to her for that. Although my understanding of who and what God is went through inevitable changes over the years, the sense of God as a supreme and loving intelligence, or Being, never really left me.

Not until I was around thirty, however, did I begin to awaken to the fact that the God, or spirit, I'd prayed to out there was really within me. That was when my prayer changed to meditation and, rather than a beseeching or a requesting, became more of a listening—a listening which led, in time, to a deep gratitude and love for life, for the movement of spirit I was beginning to feel within me.

Barbara and I have taught Adam, our son, a little about God, but not too much. We didn't want to clutter his young mind with religious ideas and dogmas. After all, we'd both learned that the energy we call "God" can be most clearly discerned when the mind is free of all such clutter.

Adam knows that God loves him, and will always take care of him. He knows that God is greater than he is, and yet he knows that God is also inside him. He understands that God speaks to him through what he has learned to call his "inner code." "Listen to your code, Adam," we used to say to him when he was young, whenever he was in doubt about what to think or do. At the same time, we've taught him that he always has a choice in life. When we ask something of him, we try and offer him at least two alternatives so that he can get to choose one for himself. This way he knows that he counts. He feels empowered. It has helped him develop good self-esteem.

Because he listens to his internal code, his communication is usually very honest and straightforward. He doesn't have a problem asking for what he wants (whereas even as an adult, I was still struggling to do that!), and he speaks from his heart. His thoughts, feelings, and actions are mostly in harmony with each other.

You educate your children, if you're conscious, so that they will grow up with a clear and strong sense of themselves, of what their gifts and talents are. You teach them how to be in the world so that they can make their way successfully in life. You teach them how to be strong, generous, and kind so that they can enjoy the quality of adult relationships that you yourself strive to have. You give them the foundational skills necessary for them to discover the answers to those basic human questions: "Who am I?" and "What do I want to do with my life?"

You take care of your children in these ways so that they can live in the world with a sense of authentic power, so that they're not held back by fear. They'll have fears of course, but if you're doing your job well, they won't be stopped by their fear. They'll forge ahead with what they really, in their hearts, want to do. They'll know that they are the source of their own experience; that they have, within them, everything they need to create the kind and quality of life they want.

Through teaching your children about personal power and creative responsibility, about how to be successful in the world—and, above all, how to contact and stay in touch with spirit, with the beauty and richness within them—you're also teaching yourself. You're reminding yourself of what is necessary for a balanced, harmonious, and fulfilling life.

Again, you see that it's not what you do in life that counts so much as the consciousness with which you do it. Educating your children to be whole human beings is the healthiest legacy you can give them. In the same way, you see that through taking care of your business and personal affairs, through staying on top of things in general—as best you can—you smooth your own way in the world.

The outer stability with which such attention provides you, makes it easier to find inner stability. Then the two come together. The age-old split between the spiritual and the material starts to be healed. Harmony and balance become a living reality for you.

Gratitude is itself an expression of joy. Remembering to give thanks whenever you feel joy is one of the surest ways to invite an even deeper joy into your life.

Chapter 18
Give Thanks

I've written of my struggle to bring my spiritual understanding into my everyday life, where it could make a difference. This struggle was most acute during the first few years following a long journey I made to Asia.

The Asian journey, especially the time in Bali, Nepal, and India, and then when I returned to my native New Zealand, where some painful childhood memories were triggered, had been a spiritual turning point for me. The experiences I went through resulted in an inner healing, something I'd been seeking all my life. I began to feel more inwardly secure, more free and trusting of the whole mysterious process of life, than I ever had before. The inner fulfillment I'd been seeking all my life—the something "more" that had always seemed to elude me in the past—had started to become a reality.

The center of my awareness, and thus my self-concept, had begun to shift out of my head—out of my intellectual understanding, my beliefs and ideas about who I was—into my body, my heart, my soul. My questions relating to who I was and what I was here for began to be answered as I found a new richness and meaning simply in *being* itself. I'd come to more of an inner silence and ease. I'd learned how to get in touch with something genuinely spiritual, if I but stopped long enough to open myself to it.

Discovering this, the spiritual truth that was at the heart of life, was a lesson in gratitude. Whenever I opened myself to spirit, to that vibrant energy of wholeness that is always here, behind creation, I felt happy and at peace. That fullness was—and is—the very essence of abundance. (The lesson, however, had actually been initiated a long time before, for even as a child I often found myself bursting forth with a prayer of thanks to God. In the innocent way that children have, I loved to thank Him for the beauty of the day, or for whatever good fortune had come to me.)

Gratitude Opens the Door to Abundance

The phrase, "My cup runneth over," took on a new and very personal meaning for me as my meditation deepened. In my most spiritually-attuned moments, my cup did indeed run over, and I felt immensely grateful for the joy of being alive, for the gift of being able to experience God's grace, the energy of spirit, of what Ramana Maharshi called the Self.

In time I discovered that gratitude itself was an important key for opening the door to the experience of inner abundance. To remember the many blessings I already had in my life helped put my mind at ease. It helped put an end to my mind's tendency to think in terms of lack and scarcity, and thus always be grasping for "more."

The blessings in my case were my largely good health (for several years I had to deal with the effects of contracting dysentery in Nepal, and that detracted somewhat from my overall well-being); the fact that I had a partner, a woman who loved me, as well as a fine son; that I had a roof over my head; and that I had regular work to support our financial needs. It was important for me to continually remember how rich, in so many ways, my life was.

Most of all, though, there was the inner richness, for I'd already begun to feel an authentic connection with the energy of spirit. When I sat to meditate, whether in my home, or in a quiet place outdoors if I was in nature, I would consciously feel a sense of inner gratitude. I'd be aware of feeling thankful. There was even a small prayer that I sometimes said, three simple words: "Thank you, Father." As I inwardly said this prayer, my body would get quiet and still, as would my mind. I'd feel all the tension and anxiety in me just drop away. Then, in the stillness and calm that followed, an exquisite energy of harmony would begin to unfold, to reveal itself to me, and I'd feel healed at every level of my being. I'd be totally renewed and revitalized, ready to face the world again.

But finding abundance in the world, finding that same sense of security materially that I experienced spiritually, presented its own problems. The deeper I went in my meditation, the more I seemed to struggle in my outer life, especially with making a success of my healing practice. I felt quite split, in fact. The truth was that I really just wanted to enjoy the bliss of meditation. I wanted to immerse myself in *being*. I didn't want to especially *do* anything, at least not anything that felt like work!

Creative activity—like writing, and exercise, and teaching workshops—always felt good to me. On the other hand, working just to make money, seeing more patients than I really wanted to see (I've always enjoyed a leisurely pace in my office, time to really connect with my patients), seemed pointless and a waste of my creative energy. After all, I knew that money was never going to fulfill me in the way that my meditation did.

Seeing the Glass Half-Full

Part of the solution to this dilemma came about one day about ten years ago, when I was having lunch with a friend, Serge Beddington-Behrens, the man who introduced me to Stephano Sabetti. Things were not going so well for me at the time and I was complaining to him about my lot in life.

Serge, who had been born into the British upper classes and was a true gentlemen, leaned forward and said, in a kindly way, "I say, old boy, it seems like we've had this conversation before. I notice you have a tendency to complain about what you don't have."

I sat up. "I do?" Even as I said it, I realized I did.

He pointed to the glass of water in front of me. "You tend to see the glass half-empty, rather than half-full."

I probably gave a sheepish grin. Serge had seen through me. "I'd like to change my attitude on that," I said. "The 'poor me' syndrome doesn't fit me very well, and it certainly doesn't feel good."

"Being grateful for what you do have, rather than always thinking about what you lack makes a difference, believe me," said Serge, with all the easy authority of one who had known only abundance and riches from the time he entered the world!

I wasn't about to admit it to him then, but some part of me was envious of Serge. I was envious of his upbringing, his aristocratic roots. His mother had been related to a Russian prince and his father, a successful businessman, had been in Winston Churchill's wartime cabinet. One of his relatives, Prince Obolensky (from whom Serge got his middle name), had been a famous rugby player for England in the early part of the century.

When Serge was young he went to Eton, Britain's most exclusive school, and then on to Cambridge University. In his early twenties he inherited an enormous sum of money. After he had spent much of it (according to him) drinking, partying, and womanizing on the Continent, he eventually came to California where he got involved in the human potential movement and ended up becoming a transformational therapist.

Why couldn't I have been born in circumstances like Serge's, a part of me wondered? How did he get to be so lucky, with all that romance, history, and wealth behind him? How come I was born into a financially struggling, semi-middle class family in suburban Auckland, New Zealand? My upbringing, my schooling, my social background seemed so mundane and uninteresting compared to Serge's. He'd had all the advantages in life—the proverbial silver spoon—and I'd had none. All Serge had to do was mention his breeding, his connections, and doors quickly and smoothly opened for him, while I'd always had to struggle, it seemed, to make any headway at all in the world.

Such was my perception at the time, anyway. Of course, if you believe in the notion of *karma*, you'll understand that we're born who we are because of what we were in our last lifetime. We come into this life with particular lessons to learn, and so we "create" the family and social circumstances in which we can best learn them. In any case, *karma* or not, the fact is that Serge, despite his aristocratic roots, had his own problems, and I certainly wasn't that disadvantaged, not compared to the majority of the people on earth.

Change Your Perception, Change Your Reality

Sitting at lunch with Serge, thinking about the differences in our backgrounds, reminded me of a past-life regression I'd done once. It was in the late Seventies. I'd met a man who specialized in taking people back into their past lives through hypnosis. I'd been referred to him by others who said that his technique really worked.

So I signed up for a session and went to his house, where I was instructed to make myself comfortable on a bed, while he sat beside me and proceeded to put me into a deeply relaxed trance. I then started to take a journey, guided by him, back through time, back before my birth, before my conception even.

After a while I found myself having what appeared to be a dream. In the dream I was living in a mud hut, not unlike a converted pig-sty, near a dirt road that made its way to a large castle on a hill. I was the youngest son in a peasant family. The era was the fourteenth or fifteenth century and the place was somewhere in France. I was dressed in rags and had a dirty face and grubby fingernails. I was standing by the fence near the road, watching some knights riding by. They were on their way to the castle, and they were all handsomely dressed in helmets and chain-mail as they rode their beautiful horses.

As I watched these knights riding haughtily past me, not even deigning to notice my existence, I felt an acute sense of resentment and injustice. Why did they have so much in their lives, so much wealth, ease, and power, while my family had to struggle in such poverty and squalor? What had they done to deserve what they had, and what had I done to deserve my circumstances? It seemed terribly,

terribly unfair and the worst of it, of course, was that I was power-less to do anything at all about it. I was only a child, after all. Yet as I watched them ride off toward the castle, I wasn't too young to notice a feeling of hopelessness and despair when I started to think about my situation in life.

When I looked back at my past I could see how this envy and resentment of others, along with a strong sense of social injustice, certainly had a place in my psychological make-up. Life did seem very unfair at times. I was aware, too, how I felt that sense of unfair-ness most acutely when I was the one who was missing out, or when others seemed to be gaining an advantage at my expense.

Over the years though, my perspective began to shift. I saw that things didn't just happen to me, even though I'd often believed that they did. I began to learn that I had a choice, that I could create dif-ferent circumstances in my life if I really wanted them, if it was important to me to do so.

As another friend of mine liked to say, "We're dealt a certain hand in life. It's up to us how we play it." He added, "And it's the way you choose to see the hand before you, that will dictate how well you play it. See it as hopeless, and it will be. Look for the promise, the potential in it, and you'll find it." In medieval France, as the son of a peasant family, my hand may not have been very promising, my choices—and my vision—may have been very limited, but this was not the case now, in twentieth century America.

That lunch with Serge reminded me that I still had a tendency at times to think of myself as a victim of circumstances. My com-plaining about what I didn't have only reinforced that tendency. Serge was right. I needed to start seeing the glass half-full, rather than half-empty. I needed to learn to be grateful for what I had, not complain about what I didn't have.

I went away from our lunch with a new attitude, and I found it made a difference. I became much more present in my practice, for example. When I looked at my appointment book, instead of worry-ing about all the empty spaces in my schedule, I consciously said a prayer of thanks for the full ones. When I was with patients, instead of being half-attentive to them while inside I was lamenting the slow afternoon I'd be facing later that day, I was fully with them.

Naturally, I was much more effective as a healing presence because of this new attitude. And I was more satisfied within myself. By focussing on the blessings I already had in my life, rather than on what was missing, I began to feel better about myself. Feeling better about myself gave me new energy and confidence. My patients, in turn, sensed my enthusiasm and my caring, and responded more positively to my work with them. As they got well, they referred others to me and my practice grew.

The inner abundance that I'd begun to feel started to manifest itself outwardly in more material prosperity. I'd begun to change the way I perceived reality, and that changed the reality.

Being Thankful for the Blessings in Your Life

In your own life, you'll find that gratitude is one of the most healing gifts of all. The more you learn to be grateful for what you have now, for the gifts and blessings that are present in your life right now, humble or meager though they may seem to be, the more you'll discover the truth behind the Biblical phrase: "To him that hath it shall be given, to him that hath not it shall be taken away."

Gratitude and an attitude of abundance creates a feeling of fullness inside you. You stop worrying and fretting about what is missing or lacking in your life, and you start being appreciative for the things that you do have. This brings about an integration of your energy. You're no longer dissipating or fragmenting it through worry or anxiety. You begin to feel more at ease within, better about yourself, stronger, more confident. In this way you start to see how gratitude is a very empowering feeling. It gets you in touch with—and helps stimulate—your own creative energy.

This is how the feeling of already *having* a sufficiency of supply, of whatever it is you need, leads to having even more. The feeling of inner abundance acts as a magnet and affects the way you think, feel, and behave, which in turn draws outer abundance to you. Conversely, when you feel inside yourself that you're missing something, then when you look outwards at your life, you see that same lack, that same scarcity. Just as success breeds success, so lack breeds lack.

Shifting your consciousness to one of gratitude, of inner abundance, may mean stopping to actually take stock of your life and circumstances. If this is something new for you, you can even do it as a written exercise. You can take a sheet of paper and write at the top, "The gifts in my life," or "The things I am grateful for." Then proceed to write down everything you can think of that enriches your life in some way, everything you have or are aware of that gives you cause to be thankful.

As you do this exercise, you'll realize that even the smallest, most humble things can give cause for gratitude. A friend you haven't heard from in a while calls you on the phone. You wake up realizing you had an exceptionally restful night's sleep. The sun suddenly comes out after it has been gloomy and overcast all morning. A piece of music you love is played on the radio. Someone says something that gives you a new idea, or that fills you with inspiration, or solves a problem you've been grappling with.

A stranger compliments you. A memory that you had long forgotten and that is particularly meaningful for you suddenly pops into your mind. A check that you hadn't expected arrives in the mail. A bill you were waiting for turns out to be less than you'd anticipated. Somebody misses an appointment and suddenly you have a whole extra hour to yourself. A bird that you've always loved—a red-tailed hawk, or a blue heron—flies by, just for your own private delight.

These are the small (or perhaps not so small, depending on how you view them) things that happen to each of us every day. By consciously acknowledging them and expressing thanks for them— whether through a prayer, a smile, or simply an attitude of inner appreciation—you reaffirm your own existence, your own beingness. You reaffirm your gratitude for the gift of life itself. And this gratitude, in turn, leads you to a deeper experience of yourself, the joy that's within you.

The Gift of the Moment at Hand

It's when you're able to sit quietly and just be appreciative for the gift of the moment itself that you're most near to your true Self. You can actually begin to taste this nearness right now, if you'd like.

Once you've finished reading this chapter, put this book down and take a few moments to be quiet and still. Let go of the thoughts in your mind—or, if you have difficulty letting them go, then don't worry about them. Focus your attention instead on your breathing. Let your breathing be deep, and as effortless as possible. Then feel yourself in your body. Let go of any holding or tension in your body.

Then take in your environment. Notice your surroundings. If there's anything of particular beauty in your awareness (and there's sure to be something that strikes you—a view perhaps, or a painting, or some flowers, or a person you care about, or an animal you love), take particular note of it. Notice your enjoyment of it. Notice how the beauty you're perceiving stirs something within you—a feeling of wholeness, of harmony and oneness.

Let all these awarenesses come together, then, into one full and flowing feeling of gratitude. Allow yourself to feel how deeply grateful you are for this moment, for the peace and the timelessness of this moment. Realize that any prayer you might want to say now would simply be a *thanking*, an acknowledgment to God for all the good things you've been graced with in your life.

When you feel these moments of inner fullness, of spiritual unity, there is nothing missing in you or in your experience. These are the most life-affirming moments. These are the moments when you're reminded of who you really are, and of what is most important to you. These are the moments when you come Home to your spiritual center.

Learn to savor these moments. Learn to be grateful for them. Take time for them at odd occasions throughout the day. Get to know your inner Self well. Learn the way Home so that you can get back there whenever you feel the need to nourish or renew yourself. Use the gift of gratitude to discover the fullness of your own being, and then let your inner fullness manifest outwardly in your life. Create something beautiful with your life. You can do it. That's why you're here.

A day will come when gratitude will be your natural state. As your enlightenment and understanding deepen and you get freer of your ego—the "me" that gets caught in judgment and comparison, that fluctuates between feeling like a victim and feeling on top of things—you'll live more spontaneously from your true nature.

You won't think in terms of "lack," or even of "abundance." You'll just live your life, take care of business, do what you love to do, and enjoy whatever the moment has to offer. Whenever you stop to think about it, you'll be aware of how deeply thankful you are.

The "great" secret is learning to let go. It's in those moments when you let go of everything in your mind—thoughts, beliefs, ideas, images, memories, dreams, hopes, and fantasies—that the healing energy of life reveals itself to you in all its beauty, immensity, and wonder.

Chapter 19
Learn to Let Go

Perhaps the hardest lesson on the journey of healing and spiritual awakening, yet the one we must all sooner or later learn, is that of letting go. The great traditions, both of the East and the West, speak of non-attachment, of surrender, of dying in order to be reborn, all of which suggest a letting go at a very deep level.

Yet when you let go, what is left? What do you find? Is there just emptiness, nothingness, meaninglessness—which is what it perhaps feels like when you contemplate the letting go of all that you hold most dear to you? Or does something else begin to arise, is there in fact the birth of something new?

There's an old Zen saying: "Now that my house has burned to the ground, I have an unobstructed view of the rising moon."

This is one of my favorite teachings from Zen, for it says so much about the true meaning of letting go. When you lose something—or someone—precious or meaningful to you, it's natural to grieve. Sometimes your grief may be deep and intense. But the more attuned you are to your true spiritual nature, the sooner the day comes when the grieving too falls away. Once again, open your eyes to the wholeness, to the pristine beauty—the rising moon—that is always here, within and around you.

The goal of Zen, and of all spiritual work, is to awaken to the wholeness that is your nature, and then to deepen your relationship with it, to learn to live in the world with it. It's to learn, as I said in the Introduction, that you're more than your body, mind and emotions, more than your personality, or the role you play in life. It's to learn that you're bigger than any fear or conflict you may experience.

It's to be in touch with something deep and meaningful within yourself, something rich and timeless that is the source of everything you are.

The Real Letting Go is an Inner Process

How many times have you read in a book with a spiritual theme that there's really nothing to attain or achieve, that you're perfect as you are, that the kingdom is within you? It's a day of great laughter and joy—in Zen it's called *kensho*, or *satori*—when you actually glimpse, for the first time, the truth of your own innate beauty and perfection.

Kensho is a taste of enlightenment, *satori* is a deeper realization of the same truth. With the former, you see it then lose it, whereas the latter changes you permanently. You actually feel, at a cellular level, your oneness with all of life. The past and future no longer have such a hold on you. The present moment becomes a shimmering, vibrant reality. You can never completely go back to your former time-bound, ego-centered consciousness.

We all experience these *kenshos*, or mini-*satoris*. On my own journey there were countless times when I found myself embroiled in some mental or emotional turmoil, and then something would happen—perhaps something as simple as a taking a deep breath—and all of a sudden the confusion would fall away, and I'd find myself in a state of clarity and ease. "What was all the fuss about?" I'd say to myself, and I'd marvel again at how simple and perfect life really is.

For me, then, this lesson of letting go has been a vital one. Each time I did let go of whatever I was holding onto internally—a belief, a resentment, an expectation—I'd feel a new sense of freedom, of lightness.

Enlightenment, I began to appreciate, was very much a feeling of lightness and expansion. It was a "lightening up." I'd heard others use the term "endarkenment" to mean the opposite of "enlightenment." It was a made-up word, of course, but an apt one. It referred to a heavy, uncomfortable, repressive state of consciousness—the unenlightened state, the state of mental and emotional contraction, of suffering, with which I, and most people, were so familiar.

Once I'd tasted the freedom and openness of enlightened awareness, of a consciousness not limited or burdened by conflicting thoughts and repetitive ideas, I naturally wanted more of it. Like the moth being drawn to the flame, I started to seek out the light. My *being* loved the feeling of expansion and space, of infinite possibility, of playful opportunity. Indeed, I haven't met a human being who didn't have, somewhere inside them, this love for freedom, for unrestrained self-expression, for play and creativity, even though outwardly they may have clung to limitation and conformity.

Letting go, then, became the way of my meditation, my spiritual practice. As I sat to meditate I'd breathe consciously, deeply, and this always brought about a letting go of tension at the physical level. This in turn helped me relax inwardly, helped me to be still, to be sensitive and aware. Then I'd notice the thoughts and ideas that I was clinging to in my mind, and I'd experiment with letting go of them. If I was particularly obsessed or worried about something, I'd make an agreement with myself. I'd tell myself that I would put the problem aside for fifteen or twenty minutes, and when my meditation was over, I could pick it back up again, if I wanted, and obsess as much as I liked.

Doing this showed me that I could let go of something I'd been holding onto, and it was okay. I discovered that the worries and problems I'd been so obsessed with really were not such a big deal after all. The more I was able to let go of them, the more I discovered that beneath the surface conflict in my mind, there was something deeper awaiting me. With each letting go, space would open up and a new insight, a new feeling, would come in. Whenever I did that experiment, then once my meditation was over, the problem—and the obsession around it—always seemed to be gone. There was just no longer any energy around it.

As you go further in your meditation there may come a point when thoughts drop away altogether—even if only for a few moments—and there is just space, clarity, and the sense of something vast. It's in these moments that your spiritual nature begins to reveal itself to you. There's a sense of infinite well-being, of the utter goodness and rightness of everything—of what, in Zen, is called the suchness of life.

The real letting go, then, is an inner process. It's the letting go of your beliefs and opinions, of the ideas and images you have about yourself that you've relied on, in the past, to sustain your ego, the "story" you've made up about your life. This is the true renunciation. In learning to let go inwardly, you get freer of the need for a self-concept, you get freer of the need to define yourself through beliefs and images. You get free of the need to have a "story" at all.

Your identity, your sense of who you are, stems more and more from *being* itself, from the direct, intuitive knowing that you're beautiful—that you're enough—as you are.

Living Out of Clarity and Freedom

With this inner renunciation, the outer things assume more perspective in your life. You're able to relate to them from clarity and freedom. You may have material riches or not, depending upon your circumstances, your fortunes, your needs, on how hard you want to work. There won't be that desperate attachment, that addictive clinging to them though, because your sense of identity won't come from outside yourself. It will come more and more from the growing knowledge of who you are at an inner, spiritual level.

Similarly, while your relationships will be important to you, because you love and care about people, there won't be the same attachment to them. You won't feel the need any longer to cling to people emotionally, or to make demands upon them. Consequently, people will enjoy being with you more. Everyone likes to feel free to be themselves when they're with others.

When someone you love leaves you, when they go away or die, you'll feel sad, of course, but the sadness will have its season. At some point, when your grieving is over, you'll again awaken to the ever-present beauty and fullness of life.

The more open and in touch you are with *being*, with your true Self, the more fully you'll feel all of your emotions. Yet even in the very moment of feeling them you'll know that you're not them. You'll be able to laugh and cry, you'll be able to get angry and sad. At the same time, you'll be able to watch yourself going through these different feelings and states, and you won't be overwhelmed by them.

Your emotions will manifest as appropriate and totally spontaneous responses to the situations and circumstances in your life. And then, once they've flowered and had their expression, they'll fall away again, and you'll be left in that state of simple clarity and openness, where the basic mood or feeling will be one of continuing wonder at the ceaselessly rich unfolding of life.

There's a natural humility that is stirred in you through this process of learning to let go. You begin to realize how beyond comprehension it all really is, this adventure we call "life." No wonder we come up with words like "God" or "Buddha-nature" to explain it all. In the end—and each moment, if you're awake to it, is both an ending and a beginning—you just have to bow down to it, and be thankful for the gift of being here.

It truly is a great and wondrous mystery, and somehow it's all exactly as it's meant to be.

Dying to the Moment

When you carry this theme of letting go to its natural conclusion, you must inevitably consider the issue of death and of dying. Some of the clearest and simplest teaching around the art of dying was given by Krishnamurti, who himself made his transition, at the age of ninety, less than ten years ago. Viewed from one perspective, his whole teaching was about learning how to die. "Die to the moment, Sir, die to the past," he would say, and it became a kind of *mantra*—not that Krishnamurti, the ultimate iconoclast, would have approved of *mantras*!—for those who sensed the importance of his message.

By dying to the past he meant the letting go of everything that you were holding onto in your mind. It was to end or negate thoughts as they arose, not allowing them to take hold and thus carry you off into conceptual or emotional states. (Of course, he was referring to ego-based thinking, the kind of psychological and emotional chatter that reinforces the "me," the sense of being a separate self, and independent entity. Krishnamurti always acknowledged and valued the role of thinking as a tool, as a function of our intelligence that was essential to both our survival and our creativity.)

When you were able to do this, he would say, when you were able to die to each moment, then you'd be no longer afraid of death itself. In facing your own psychological death throughout the day—the ending of the "me" and all that it clings to—you would understand, intuitively, that there really is no death, only the eternal current of life, of creation, of *being*.

A Story about Krishnamurti

In regard to this letting go, I remember a story about Krishnamurti related to me by my friend, Erich Schiffmann, who had taught yoga for five years at Brockwood Park, Krishnamurti's school in England. Apparently there were only two television sets in the entire school: one in Krishnamurti's room—he loved to watch T.V., with *Kojak* and *Monty Python* being among his favorite programs—and the other in the school common room.

Because there were a number of channels to choose from on the British television network, a T.V. committee had been formed, composed of members of the staff and student body. It was their job to select the programs to be viewed. One evening, the film *The Godfather* was due to be shown. A lot of the students, and probably a few staff too, wanted to watch this highly-acclaimed movie, but it was voted down. "Too violent and not in keeping with the kind of sensitive, enlightened attitude we're trying to foster at this school," was the general feeling of the committee, if not their actual statement. So the decision was made to watch something else on another channel.

The next morning everyone was assembling in the dining-room for breakfast when Krishnamurti strode in in his usual erect and highly alert way.

"Did you watch *The Godfather* last night?" he queried a group of students near him. "Wonderful movie, wonderful!"

The students looked at him in shock. "No, the committee voted against it," one of the students said, while the others simply gaped, and probably inwardly cursed themselves for the decision that had been made. If it was okay for the great man himself to watch it, surely they could have too. "We thought it was too violent, the wrong kind of thing to put into our minds."

"Nonsense," Krishnamurti snorted, making a dismissive gesture with his hand. Then his voice softened a little and he looked at the gathering audience of students and staff around him. "Don't you see?" he said, in that kind, compassionate way he had. "You watch it, and then you *drop* it."

You watch it and then you drop it. This was one of the key themes in Krishnamurti's whole teaching. He wasn't against movies, or entertainment, or sex, or sports, or having fun. For him, life was a gift, a blessing, and it was definitely to be lived. The main thing was that you didn't harm anyone—or yourself—through your actions; that you didn't get so lost in the pursuit of pleasure that you missed the true beauty in life, because it was the sense of beauty, of there being something timeless, that gave rise to compassion, to love. And it was only love that would heal the suffering that was everywhere.

The secret was to not hold onto anything in your mind. It was to let go of an experience as soon as it was over. It was to die completely to what had gone before so that you could experience something totally new and fresh in the present.

Facing Death Itself

To learn the real meaning and value of letting go, sometimes we need the actual experience of facing death itself. There have been a number of occasions in my own life when I directly confronted my own fear of death, when I actually thought that I was in all likelihood going to die. Each of them, in their own way, helped me get freer of the various illusions I was attached to, the beliefs that reinforced my self-concept. In getting free, I gradually came upon a more authentic experience of my true Self, and was more able to face my fear of dying the next time it came around.

The first time I confronted death was in Vietnam, where I was a young artillery officer, part of a small New Zealand unit that was attached to an Australian brigade. Our fire base was under attack from a Viet Cong force, and the cry came out over our Command Post loudspeaker, "Watch the wire! They're coming through the wire!" Our barbed wire perimeter was only fifty meters from my bunker and I remember standing and frantically trying to cock my automatic pistol, convinced that we were about to be overrun by a horde of charging, screaming Viet Cong. I was terrified. Scenes from my life flashed before me. I didn't feel ready to die at all—I was only twenty years old—and yet the awful truth struck me that, ready or not, it was suddenly about to happen.

As it turned out, the ground attack didn't come at our perimeter, but on the other side of the fire base. With support from American helicopter gunships and our superior firepower, the small Viet Cong force was eventually beaten back. Nevertheless, we'd taken casualties. I'd heard an Australian soldier moaning in pain only a short distance from our unit. He'd been sleeping in an armored personnel carrier that had been struck by a rocket-propelled grenade. It pierced the thin armor of the APC and sent flakes of hot metal spinning around inside the small compartment, a nightmarish inferno that had so badly wounded the poor soldier he later died.

The next morning, at dawn, an hour or two after the fighting stopped, I went over to the other perimeter to inspect the breach that had been made in the wire. I had my first view ever of death, the bodies of four Viet Cong. They were gray, ashen in the morning light. One of them had half his head and jaw shot away, probably by a .50 caliber machine gun bullet. The impact had scooped his brain out, so that what was left of his head looked like an empty, broken gourd with a few tufts of black hair on it. Another man, who was very young—just a boy, really—had an innocent, unmarked face, a shocked expression in his eyes. His black fatigue shirt was pulled up and twisted around his body, and there were several bullet holes in his side—smooth, dark punctures that didn't look all that nasty. Yet they'd killed him.

I remember looking at these bodies in amazement and thinking that, just a few hours before, they had been living, moving, breathing human beings just like me. And the only difference between us now was this thing called life, the animating force of consciousness (although I wouldn't have used the word "consciousness" in those days). I was still standing there, still breathing, still able to think, to sense, to feel, and they weren't.

Like our first sexual experience, or our first enlightenment, when we realize that Reality is much more than we'd ever imagined it to be, seeing a dead human being for the first time—especially when the death is so sudden and violent—isn't something we forget. It's a powerful rite of passage. It both teaches us about the preciousness of life, and awakens us to the ever-present fact of our own mortality. It reminds us of how thin the veil between life and death really is. To stare death in the face is to receive one of the most compelling lessons of all in the art of letting go.

When I stood there that morning in Vietnam after our base was attacked and I'd thought I was going to die, and looked down on those four dead bodies, something in me let go. I lost my innocence, my unquestioning belief that no real harm could ever befall me, and that I would somehow live forever. Now I knew for certain that one day I was going to die. I stopped taking my life quite so much for granted.

The second occasion when I came face-to-face with my own mortality was the health crisis I went through during chiropractic school. This was the event I referred to at the beginning of this book, and that started me on my spiritual journey. During the worst times of this period in my life, I'd be lying in bed at night, struggling to breathe, to get free of the constriction in my chest. I would fight the impulse to fall asleep. I was afraid that if I did let go, I'd no longer have conscious control over my breathing, and that I'd therefore stop breathing and die.

And yet even during the times of the greatest fear, something in me knew that if I could only let go of my control, my fear, and just relax and fall asleep, I'd both be free of the problem I was having, and I'd break through into a new level of consciousness. I'd already begun reading about enlightenment, and even then, novice that I was in matters of the heart and spirit, I sensed that somehow I was being challenged to face my true Self.

But I wasn't ready to look at my fear—and I was at least clear enough to acknowledge that I wasn't ready. I still had a very strong attachment to my self-identity, and my self-identity was very much linked to my bodily well-being. If being enlightened meant staying with my fear and somehow surrendering to it, I would remain, at least for the time being, unenlightened. There was no way I was ready to confront that degree of letting go. Whenever the fear got too much for me at night, I continued to do what I'd done right from the beginning: I'd lurch out of bed and try escape from it. I'd move, walk, think, read, do anything I could to distract myself from it, until it passed.

After six months or so of yoga, meditation and learning to slow down, the symptoms that I was having began to disappear, and with it the fear. Once in a while I'd have a flashback that would make me anxious, but I was finally beginning to be more at ease within myself. I'd begun to let go of the old, rigid "me." I was loosening up somewhat. I was going through—albeit slowly—an inner transformation.

Eight years after that experience at chiropractic school, I found myself sitting cross-legged on a beach in Bali, watching the sunset and reflecting on my fears around commitment, especially concerning the relationship I was in. I had resolved to sit there on the beach until I'd gained some insight into the matter, because it was an old issue for me. I'd always had a problem with commitment. It was time to take a close look at why it continued to come up.

The experience on the beach turned out to be a kind of completion for me. It marked a completion of the journey that had started back at chiropractic school, when I had first intuited that, if I could but summon up the courage to face my fear of death head-on, I might be a freer person, free in the way I'd always wanted to be.

After an hour or so of sitting on the beach, wrestling with my issues around commitment, my fear of entrapment, of losing my self by becoming too enmeshed in the emotional reality of another person, a motorcycle came by. Local Balinese boys and Australian surfers often rode on the beach. The motorcycle passed below me, on the hard sand near the water-line. It seemed to create a tremor in the ground because my body started to shake, to vibrate.

As I watched its red tail-light disappear into the night, I felt the vibration travel up my back and around into my chest. Suddenly, I realized that it wasn't the ground that was moving, but me. I was having a *kundalini* experience of some kind. The pressure in my chest intensified. My breathing became difficult. My body stiffened and I felt a rising panic, just as I had during those months at chiropractic school when I was afraid to fall asleep at night.

All my old anxiety was re-stimulated. My heart pounded furiously as I struggled to breathe, fighting the powerful energy that was gripping me from inside. Afraid that if I sat there any longer I'd lose consciousness, I started to get up. I told myself that if I just ran down the beach as fast as I could, I'd be able to release whatever the energy was, and shake my fear away. But then I remembered something I'd said to myself earlier: I'd made an agreement with myself to stay there, on the beach, until I learned something about commitment. I'd made a commitment to finding out about commitment! Was I going to run now, as I'd always done?

Then I remembered something else, something I'd learned in recent years that would have helped me get through that stressful episode in chiropractic school, had I known about. It was the technique which I described in the second chapter of this book, one of the most important transformational tools of all.

I remembered to *breathe*.

I took a slow, deep breath. I breathed all the way into my fear. I paused, and breathed again. Almost immediately, I felt a lessening of tension. As I continued to breathe, the rigidity and fear in my body began to let go. The intense energy subsided, gave way to a new feeling, an energy that was much lighter, smoother. I felt a sense of well-being begin to course through my body. I remember sighing with gratitude. I'd done something I'd not been able to do during that time of the stress eight years before: I'd faced my fear of death, of suffocation, and I'd come out safely on the other side—not just safe, but stronger and more self-assured.

There were times after that experience in Bali when I'd find myself feeling the contracting energy of fear again, but now I knew what to do. I discovered that if I just remembered to breathe—and to be totally present in my body, with my experience—then I could breathe my way through anything.

You, too, will be called upon at some time to face your fear of dying, of suffocation, if you haven't already done so. You can be sure of that. This was one of the Buddha's most important teachings—that before a man or woman could become enlightened, he or she had to face the three specters of sickness, old age, and death. The beautiful thing about meditation, about learning to let go of whatever it is you're holding onto, is that you face the reality of death in each moment. In dying to the moment in this way, you gradually learn that death is not such a big thing, it's not something to be feared.

By going through these little deaths constantly throughout the day, dropping thoughts and memories as they arise—enjoying them if you want, by all means, but not clinging to them too tightly, or making too big a thing out of them—you'll find yourself more at ease in the present. You'll find yourself much less tense, much less anxious.

The world's religions give us a variety of accounts of what happens after death, yet if we're honest with ourselves, none of us really knows. This is why the prospect of dying, especially when we still enjoying living, can be so frightening. (Admittedly, for some people—those afflicted with great pain or suffering—death is sometimes welcomed as a release.) But what the inner spiritual journey does for us, this learning to let go of all that we hold onto inwardly, is that it teaches us to live without fear of life or death.

We no longer think or worry about dying, in other words, because we're so fully alive in the present. We truly do die, psychologically, to each moment. And then, when the moment of physical death does come, as it inevitably will, we'll face it with the same quality of presence, openness, and trust that we've learned to bring to every other moment in our lives.

Not Holding onto Anything

The more you let go, the more you come upon the energy of your true Self, the wisdom, love, and power within you. As you learn to live more in freedom, the past will become less and less real to you.

Someone will mention some time or event from the past, or you'll look at a photograph or think of something that happened once, and it will seem like another incarnation to you, a previous lifetime.

You'll realize that the past is to be honored, but it's not something to cling to, like some psychological lifeboat. Nor will you obsess about the future. Plans have to be made, yes, and goals set, but as you learn to let go of the kind of grasping that reinforces the insecure "I," or ego, you'll find it easier to hold the future in perspective too. In the end, the feeling of being alive, creative, and free in the present will be far more important to you than the memory of what has been, or the elusive promise of what is yet to come.

Nor will you try to hold onto the peace you find, nor to the joy or bliss that you'll begin to experience with increasing frequency. Indeed, the less you hold on, the more these feelings will be there. You'll see the folly of trying to hold onto, or seek out, any state. It's the ego that wants to cling, to grasp. This is how it survives and maintains its hold over you. This is how the ego, with all its fears and worries, exercises its grip on your being, your Self, and blocks your creative potential.

As you become more adept at letting go, all these things will become more evident to you, and the way itself will be easier. You'll still continue to be challenged, you'll still have problems, and times when you don't feel well, or when you don't know what to do, but you won't be so attached to these passing states of doubt and conflict. You'll see them more and more for what they are—aspects of the human condition, the moods, feelings and behaviors to which we all fall prey at times. You'll let go of your need to judge them negatively, and you'll just breathe your way through them, always knowing that, "This too shall pass."

Letting Go of the Need to Understand

A final note: the very fact that you're reading this book indicates that you have a commitment to understanding your own process and to gaining a deeper feeling for what your life is all about, so that you can heal your own suffering and enjoy a happier and more fulfilling existence.

Any understanding you gain will inevitably translate itself into certain ideas, beliefs, or concepts. If your understanding is not yet embodied—that is to say, if it doesn't stem from your direct, personal experience—it will tend to remain in the realm of intellectual understanding.

Intellectual understanding, while at first stimulating and even exciting, eventually becomes tiresome if it doesn't have some experiential substance behind it. Words alone, while they may succeed in partially describing the flower, can never really give you the perfume you're seeking. Sooner or later words lose their freshness, their impact, their ability to move and inspire you. Only with a direct experience of the flower, of truth itself, can you smell the fragrance. It's Rumi all over again. You have to taste in order to know.

This is why one of the most important lessons in letting go—and one of the most freeing—is learning to let go of the need to interpret, to conceptually understand your experience. The more you're able to let go of the words, beliefs, and theories, the more you'll find yourself in pure, open experience. And in that openness, in the living, breathing realm of what you're actually *experiencing*, new sensations and feelings will be felt, new perceptions gained, new insights and awarenesses will arise.

The mind, of course, wants to understand. It wants to have everything figured out. That's its nature. In order to have a contented, conflict-free mind, it's necessary to have things figured out. That's why we embark on our quest in the first place—to seek answers to those questions that trouble us, that sometimes even torment us!

This is where teachings that are true, that are accurate reflections of the reality they are attempting to describe, can be of such a big help. As Jean Klein taught me, true communication arises out of silence, and leads back into it. When you're deeply sensitive to what you're feeling, you can speak the truth about it. Similarly, when you hear the truth spoken to you, it resonates within you and dissolves, ultimately, in silence. It brings you back into your heart, to the feeling of love.

As you seek answers to your most pressing questions, seek them with your whole heart and mind, you'll find that the answers will come more quickly when you let go of analytical thinking and give up trying to "figure out" everything. Eventually things will begin to fall naturally into place. As you let go of your need to understand, you'll become quieter and more at ease within. You'll be more aware, more present.

Sooner or later, Reality—the innate beauty and joy of life—will reveal itself to you, if only for a moment. And then, in that moment, you'll understand. You'll know everything you need to know. You'll know what matters most. You'll appreciate Ramana Maharshi's statement that the highest truth is to be found in silence. It is the great teacher. It is the true power.

In that silence, you'll discover, lies the peace that is beyond all understanding.

Once you've made the choice to awaken, to become fully conscious, then the way to live your life becomes clear. All the other choices you need to make will flow out of that.

Chapter 20
Choose!

At the end of the Introduction to this book, I wrote, "If you choose the path of consciousness and keep listening to your heart, keep bringing your attention back to the present, you'll come upon that energy, I promise."

We're now nearing the end of the book itself. In this, the next-to-last chapter, I want to explore more fully the subject of choice, which I touched on in Chapter Fifteen—Know What You Want. As I said in the Introduction, "You awaken the healing energy within you through your determination to find it. It is, in the end, a choice you make."

Yes, the choice as to what you do with your life, and where you put your attention, is yours. This can be a rather intimidating proposition, or an immensely liberating one, depending on how you view it. Choice doesn't only mean freedom, it also implies responsibility. While most of us want the freedom, not all of us are ready or willing to assume the responsibility.

Before I talk about the power of choice, let me say more about this promise I've made to you—that you'll awaken the healing energy within you, if your determination is but strong enough. You might be wondering how I can make such a promise. How can I be so sure, you may be asking yourself? What proof or grounds do I have in order to justify my conviction? Many of you reading these pages will already have at least a feel for what I'm saying. You'll have had a taste of what in Zen is called your "Buddha-mind." You'll have touched enough of those moments of luminous peace and clarity to know, beyond any doubt, that they're real.

There are, however, many people—you may or may not be among them—who don't yet trust this. You may intellectually understand that the well-being you seek is within you, but perhaps you don't yet have a real feeling for it. Your inner experience, not to mention the outer circumstances in your life, may be so conflict-ridden or unfulfilling at this time that you simply can't believe that you are, in your natural state, a radiant and loving human being.

If this is the way you feel, then don't despair. The truth is, none of us really trusts our inner Self very much until we have a more authentic connection with it. We still fall prey to the pull of our ego, of self-will, whenever something seductive—or threatening—passes in front of us.

If we're feeling empty or unhappy inside, and there's a chance to do something stimulating and diverting (even when we know we're going to have to eventually face our emptiness), we nevertheless go ahead and do it. When encountering a conflict, a problem, a crisis, instead of getting quiet and still and easing into meditation for our guidance, our answer, we still tend to hunt—often frantically!—for ego-based solutions.

Forgetting who we really are, we look outward at the world, at the confusing flux of events and circumstances, and take them to be real. We try to juggle the situations in our outer life in order to give ourselves some measure of peace and happiness within. In the end though, we always end up frustrated. We're always left grasping for "more."

Learning to Trust

What is it, then, that brings us to the place where we finally begin to trust the movement of spirit within us?

The process often begins with trusting someone on the outside first, someone who seems to know what they're talking about— someone who is established, to some degree, in that energy. Jean Klein gives the example of asking someone for directions to a particular street. As you listen to the person giving directions, you're also—at least unconsciously—sizing them up. You're asking yourself, "Is this person trustworthy?" Most of the time, of course, we do trust the person who is giving us directions. We follow the directions they gave us and, all going well, we end up where we wanted to be.

Sometimes the directions are incorrect, however, and they don't bring us to our desired goal. We trusted the wrong person! Either they misled us or, more likely, they just didn't have the right information. In that case, there's nothing to do but go and seek other directions—this time from someone whom, we hope, knows what he or she is talking about.

In spiritual matters it's all too easy, unfortunately, to be misguided—and, as a result, to make poor choices. I wrote of this in an earlier chapter when I talked about *gurus* and teachers who, in spite of an enlightened understanding of some aspects of life, or the ability to wield certain powers and even transmit spiritual energy, are still trapped by their egos. Whenever the ego gets involved you can be sure that the teacher has his or her own best interests at heart, not those of the student.

How do you tell, then? How do you tell a good teacher from one who is not good? There's a simple answer: you trust the teacher who says that what you're seeking is within you and who, at the same time, gives you complete freedom to listen or not listen to their teaching. If you don't feel any sense of being coerced, seduced, or made to do anything against your own will or better judgment, then you can probably learn something from that teacher without getting hurt in the process.

So you listen to the instructions of the teacher for finding your way back Home, to the source of energy within. You try whatever practices or techniques are recommended to see how they work for you. In the same way, I'm inviting you to trust that what I'm saying is true. I've given you, in these twenty chapters, some directions for discovering the light and the beauty that I know, without any doubt, is there inside you. I'm passing on to you much of what has been given to me by my teachers, though from the perspective of my own understanding and experience.

The rest is up to you. No teacher can go where you need to go. I certainly can't do it for you. Only you can uncover the spiritual treasure that's within you. Indeed, that's the real meaning of the word guru. The true guru (or "dispeller of darkness" as it translates from Sanskrit) is you. Spell the word out and you'll see what I mean: G-U-R-U. *Gee, You Are You*!

An Experience of Initiation

Let me share a personal story which may help illustrate what I've been saying. A few years after I'd begun to meditate and do yoga, I met Erich Schiffmann. He was, at first, simply my yoga teacher, and then we became friends, travelers together on the spiritual path. One day I was meditating with Erich after a strenuous session of yoga, and I happened to open my eyes and look at him. His eyes were closed, his gaze fixed on some inner plane. I could tell from the evenness of his breathing and the energy of peace and calmness that he exuded, that whatever he was in touch with, it was very blissful.

This was a time when my own connection to that inner bliss was still tenuous. I was acquiring a lot of ideas and information about consciousness and inner peace but it was still mostly "head" stuff. I didn't have much direct experience of it. I could usually only feel it if all the circumstances in my life were harmonious, and there was nothing troubling me. Nevertheless, I trusted it was there. I trusted Krishnamurti and the other teachers who told me, through their books and their spoken words, that there was indeed something timeless, something beautiful in life, and it was within me.

I remember looking at Erich and feeling a stab of envy. He was obviously experiencing something real within himself, and I wished I could be there with him. I wished I could share it with him. I almost broke the silence in the room to ask him if he'd describe what he was experiencing, but I didn't want to disturb him.

And then, as if by magic—or Grace!—something stirred in me. I heard the words, "You can't be there, where he is. But if you get really quiet and still and go inside yourself, maybe you can find the same place within you." The voice that spoke to me was of course my intuition, my higher Self—an echo of wisdom that had been given to me in the past, and that only now I was ready to hear.

So I closed my eyes again, and got very quiet. I began to slow down my breathing, and started to tune in to the stillness in the room. Soon I became aware of how peaceful everything was, and then I noticed that the peace I was feeling was in me. I felt it as a gentle fullness, an exquisite current of energy that flowed softly through me, making every cell of my body tingle and vibrate with aliveness and joy. I felt healed, renewed. Now there was no longer any doubt. I felt totally free.

Some time later, I opened my eyes, just as Erich opened his. We looked at each other and smiled, and then we both threw our heads back and burst into laughter, the kind of happy, satisfied laughter that can't be stopped, that bubbles up and spills over all by itself.

Neither of us had to say anything. Erich, especially, wasn't one for excess words. But we both knew. We were telepathically connected. What a treat it was to be able to experience that quality of spiritual union with another person, a friend! I realized then that I'd had an initiation from Erich, whether he'd consciously transmitted his energy to me or not.

I put my hands together in gratitude for the gift that his being, his presence, had given me. He saluted back. "*Namaste*," he said with a grin.

The Power of Conscious Choice

It's time now to begin asking: What do I choose for myself? How serious am I about my spiritual awakening? Given the choices I've made up until now and the results they have brought me, what choice am I going to make for the future? Is there something I need or want to choose differently? What choice, or choices, can I make that will bring me the greatest chance for happiness and fulfillment in my life?

Recognizing the power of choice is one of the last of the tools I'll share with you in this book. We began with the need for looking within, and then examined the healing power of deep, conscious breathing—how slowing down the breath helps move you into that place where you're naturally meditating, just as I described it happening in my experience with Erich.

We come now to the power of choice because it represents, in a way, the key to all the other tools and techniques offered in this book. None of them will work for you, none of them will be of any use to you, unless you *choose* to apply them, unless you choose to at least explore them, play with them, try them out and see what relevance or meaning they may have for you.

Do you know, for instance, that the word "intelligent" comes from the Latin, *intellegere*, which literally means, to understand, or to choose between? To live intelligently is to exercise the power of conscious choice in your life. It's to be able to choose wisely, intelligently, based on your understanding of what's in your best interests.

It's having the capacity to choose those options, or courses of action, which will best serve your own—and therefore, others'—well-being.

Being True to Yourself

Let me say more about how others are served when you're being true to yourself. At first glance, the notion of really taking care of yourself and your own needs first can sound selfish and narcissistic. Yet there's great wisdom behind it. Consider these famous lines from Shakespeare's *Hamlet*:

> *This above all: to thine own self be true,*
> *And it must follow, as the night the day,*
> *Thou canst not then be false to any man.*

When you're being true to yourself, listening to your heart, your inner voice, there's an integration, a gathering of energy that happens. You're no longer fighting yourself, you're no longer divided or torn apart by doubt, or conflict. Instead, you're on purpose, on target. In those moments when you're being true to yourself, you know who you are and what you're about. There's a power and a rightness to this knowing.

This kind of certainty comes from a deep inner place. It's different from arrogance, which is a defense of the mind, the ego. It's a certainty that is immensely attractive to people. Few of us have it all the time, but most of us would like more of it. I know that the individuals I've been drawn to over the years, including those who've become my teachers, displayed this quality of being true to themselves to the highest degree. They had an inner knowing and strength that I lacked, and that I desperately wanted for myself. They didn't need approval, never looked for it, and yet they received lots of it.

Contrast this with the experience of people who, out of their insecurity, put on a mask or act in other less-than-authentic ways in order to obtain approval. They rarely get the approval they seek, and inevitably end up more unhappy than they were in the first place. Nobody wants to be around people who are phony (unless it's someone who is playing the same game).

In those moments when I was in touch with my own truth, with that place of certainty within me, I realized that I'd found what I'd been looking for all my life. The experience of being truly myself was so energizing that I naturally wanted more of it. The healing I was seeking, I realized, was precisely this quality of being in touch with my true self, my feelings, my heart's needs and desires, and honoring them.

Once I knew this (and I needed to be reminded of it constantly—and still do!), then the way was clear. I knew what my life was about. I knew what I was here for. Knowing this primary choice or direction made all the other, lesser choices—the inevitable forks in the road along life's journey—somewhat easier.

What does it mean to be true to yourself? How do you go about it? How do you accomplish it? Directly or indirectly, that's what this whole book has been about. As you experiment with the various tools and approaches to self-discovery I've shared with you, you'll find out what is true for you.

As you awaken more to your own essence, the current of aliveness, of spirit, that is uniquely yours, you'll find out what has meaning for you, and what doesn't. You'll be more in touch with your real needs. You'll know yourself better, and you'll trust yourself more.

The Art of Making the Right Choice

Of all the paths leading to self-discovery, learning to make conscious choices is definitely one of the most empowering. How do you make a conscious choice? You listen, or feel, for what is most true for you, most right for you, and then you honor that. You make a decision and you follow through.

If you listen to your inner voice, to what your heart and gut are saying, you always know how you're feeling in any given moment. Your body will give you feedback. When you're on target, you'll feel it as a "click," as a sense of rightness and knowing in all your cells. To honor that feeling—to do, in essence, what *feels* most right in that moment—is to make the choice to be true to yourself.

Sometimes the information that comes through as you listen, as you tune in to spirit, isn't very clear. Perhaps the feelings you're experiencing are vague. Your body may be giving mixed signals. They don't meld together into any clearly discernible shape or pattern. Or maybe you're just feeling downright uncertain, confused even, so that you have no idea at all of what, if any, choice you ought to make.

When the direction is unclear, you wait. This is the most common-sense approach. For years now, one of my most reliable maxims, one of those little "keys," or bits of self-talk that have proven their value over time, has been the one that says, "If in doubt, leave it out." In other words, if you don't know what to do, it's usually best not to do anything. However, this doesn't mean you then go to sleep, or spend the rest of your life being passive and refusing to make choices!

Remember, no choice is still a choice. In this kind of situation, where the direction is not sufficiently clear for you to make an intelligent choice, you're choosing to wait, to be patient until you get more insight as to what your best option is. The element of timing is often at work here. Part of maturity, of being attuned to a deeper harmony, or rhythm in life, is knowing that there really is a proper time, a season, for everything. It's knowing that sometimes it's appropriate to act, and sometimes not—just as sometimes a certain response or behavior is appropriate, and at other times it's not.

Of course, there's also the saying, "Don't just sit there, do something!" Sometimes action is demanded, a response of some kind is called for, whether you feel ready to respond or not, whether the timing is favorable or not. There are occasions when events and circumstances will accelerate beyond your control, and you're required to jump, leap into the abyss, take a chance.

If you find yourself confronted with a situation like this, then even though you may not have all the information you'd ideally like to have before you make your choice, you go with what you have. This is where the choice you make has an element of risk to it. You make the best possible choice under the circumstances, and take the risk—and trust that, if you make a mistake, you'll get an opportunity to choose differently later. As you always do.

There are No Guarantees

When I look back at my own life I can honestly say that I've never made a wrong choice. I've made poor choices, errors in judgment, mistakes—plenty!—but I don't feel I've ever made a "wrong" choice. It seems that my choices around career, relationships, places I've lived, traveling, education, money, and time management, have all played a part in bringing me to the understanding I now have.

This is not just a metaphysical explanation. Had I made better choices at certain points in my life, the path might have been easier for me. I didn't do it "perfectly" and, based on my experience, I probably never will. I think it's admirable to seek perfection in our circumstances, if by perfection we mean total harmony and order, everything falling into place without any hitches or problems. Certainly, it's to be welcomed when everything does work flawlessly.

Inevitably though, choosing always involves the element of risk. There are few, if any, guarantees in life. When John Lennon sings, "Life is what happens to you while you're busy making other plans," there's a lot of street wisdom behind his words. It's the wisdom that comes from knowing no matter how prepared you are, no matter how well you think you have chosen—or acted—things can still go awry. Life can still throw a curve ball at you.

Yet it's through risking, through having the courage to make new, different or difficult choices, that you grow. When you keep making the same unproductive or unfulfilling choices over and over again, you remain stuck in what is essentially a negative pattern of behavior. You don't get to experience your full creative potential, you don't get to try out and express other dimensions of yourself. You don't get to find out what your capabilities really are.

As you practice making new and more conscious choices, choices designed to further, or better serve, your well-being, you'll come to the realization of the truth behind Shakespeare's words: that the only way you can be happy in life is by being true to yourself.

Honoring the Call of Your True Self

Being true to yourself is how you serve others. You show them, through the example of your own conduct, how they can be true to *them*selves. You show them the way to the only happiness that can be counted on: the happiness that comes from within, that doesn't depend on outside events or circumstances, and that can't be taken away by anything or anyone. From this perspective, being true to yourself is one of the highest forms of service you can render anyone.

As you deepen your practice of making conscious choices—"Do I choose this, or do I choose *that*?"—you'll eventually come more and more to the place where you see that there's only one choice. You'll discover that you can only choose that which is healing, that which serves your own—and, therefore, others'—highest truth, or well-being. This is what Krishnamurti meant when he talked about choice and how, when you live with integrity, there is really no choice.

For it's the ego, or personal will, that makes choices and decides between "this" or "that," based upon its conditioned belief or expectation about what will gratify its needs and desires. The more you connect with the healing energy within you, with your higher Self, the less you live from your ego.

Rather than viewing your circumstances and your problems from the limited, biased perspective of an insecure ego, you begin to see life from your wholeness—from what Jean Klein calls your global awareness, your Home ground. Instead of choosing from need or lack, from trying to grasp or clutch at that which you hope will give you the feeling of security you need—which is the ego's way—you choose from abundance. Because you actually feel that connection to your true nature, you're already nourished, full, satisfied. Even in those times when you don't particularly feel it, you remember what is true, you remember who you are, and you do your best to live from that truth.

So the most important choice is to first find, and then honor, the call of your inner Self. This is why I urge you to choose the healing path. It's the most intelligent choice. When you live with a global perspective, all your intelligence becomes available. The more you're in your wholeness, your natural awareness, the more access you have to both your intuition and your powers of logic and reason.

The beauty of living this way is that during those times when things are not working out on the material plane, when your fortunes are in a downward trend, for whatever reason, you still have yourself.

You still have that source of energy within you, with all its power to bring about something new in your life.

Commitment Requires that You Make a Choice

One of my favorite quotes from Krishnamurti, words I wrote many years ago in my journal, and which continue to inspire me and remind me that I am surely on the right path, is:

> *When you live with this awareness, this sensitivity, life has an astonishing way of taking care of you, because there is no taking care on your part. Life carries you where it will because you're part of itself. Then there is no problem of security, of what people say or do not say, and that is the beauty of life.*

When you listen carefully to Krishnamurti's words, you begin to understand for yourself why spiritual awakening really is the ultimate cure for human suffering. You begin to realize why it's so necessary for each of us to open up to our true nature, to the love and joy—the creative energy—that's within each of us.

After all, the more of us there are who continue to deepen and expand our realization through learning to bring what we know into every facet of our daily life, the more the "ultimate cure" will be available to the rest of humanity. And what a difference that will make in our world!

Make the choice, then, to live with awareness and sensitivity. Find out who you really are. Look for that energy, that fire, that light within you. Get as close as you can to it, become one with it, and you'll find that all the other choices you need to make during the course of your lifetime will fall into place. They will become clearer and clearer, easier and easier. You'll let go of what is nonessential and unnecessary, in your life, and you'll find yourself being focussed and committed in a way you had perhaps never dreamed was possible.

Choice precedes commitment. This is why many of us have so much trouble around commitment. You can't commit yourself wholeheartedly to anything you haven't chosen wholeheartedly. You can't commit yourself to something—an endeavor, a project, a relationship—unless it *feels* right to you. To the degree the project or person doesn't feel right, to the degree the situation or person isn't really what you want, what you're looking for, to that degree will you be uncommitted.

In the end, you'll discover that there's only one thing in this life that you can be fully and wholeheartedly committed to, and that is the *truth*—the truth as it manifests in you, the truth as you experience it and know it. Many people get caught up in deceptions, lies, and dishonesty, but no one ever really enjoys it. No one can ever be wholly committed to such a way of living. By definition, to be dishonest is to withhold something, to pull back from revealing all. It's to put a damper on our aliveness. It's to repress our true nature.

It's to be less than who we really are.

Getting Off the Fence

Until we're committed to our highest well-being, we risk remaining on the fence. We'll continue to vacillate between this choice or that, this option or that one, and we'll be forever dissatisfied. Sitting on the fence is an extremely uncomfortable place to be. The sharp points of those pickets jab us in the most tender parts of our anatomy!

However, there's one good thing about sitting on the fence. If we sit there long enough and really pay attention to how such a way of living and being feels, we'll get so uncomfortable that sooner or later we'll do something about it! We may choose to get off the fence. We may choose to do something different, to see if we can find a better way. That's a very good start.

The more you choose well-being, the more you'll find yourself naturally committed to the healing path. It'll become less of a struggle to do what is right, to do what serves your best interests. You'll eventually get so sick of the other way of living, of conflict and disharmony in your life, that you'll do something about it. Either the feeling of acute frustration, the stress of such a way of living, or illness itself (for illness is a big stick), will compel you to make a move.

It's when the need for a more balanced life becomes very strong within you, that your ego will diminish. You'll be less and less interested in giving energy to the beliefs and expectations, the fears and judgments that support it and help it maintain its hold over you. Your fear of not really living, of wasting your life, will become stronger than the fear of stepping out, of risking.

You'll start to listen more to the real call—the voice of your soul—within you. You'll get quieter within. You'll find yourself thinking and speaking less, so that you can be open to the deeper wisdom. You'll naturally begin to choose what is most right for you. All your energies will begin to come together. You'll be living with a renewed sense of purpose, of wonder, of passion. You'll be willing to take risks.

You'll feel reborn. This feeling of rebirth is one of the best feelings there is, because now you're conscious, now you have vision and wisdom. You're no longer a helpless victim. To be reborn spiritually in this way is to be given a whole new lease on life. And it's happening because you chose it.

You chose to do something differently, and so something different is happening.

Discover your true spiritual identity, and you'll find the peace, love, and happiness you've been seeking.

Chapter 21
Remember Who You Are

As you go further on your healing journey, you'll begin to realize with increasing certainty that your real nature is spirit, God, consciousness. In those moments when you find yourself simply present, quiet, at peace, you'll feel the current of harmony that is underneath all life, that is the very source and pulse of creation. You'll feel it in your body as aliveness and well-being. You'll feel it in your mind as a luminous quality of clarity and openness. You'll feel it in your heart as unity, or oneness with all life—and with it, a welling up of gratitude, love, and affection.

What you feel may not be easy to put into words, but that won't matter. Somehow, at some level, you'll realize that you and it—the feeling—are One. The gap between you and the peace you're experiencing will tend to disappear. You'll no longer cling to concepts, words, and ideas that tend to separate you from the beauty and fullness of the moment. You'll realize with more and more certainty that you are that beauty, and that you're loved by life, by God.

The essence of the healing energy I've been talking about throughout this book is love. It's love that will heal you of your own pain and suffering. It's love that will inspire you to live your life in a way that is true for you, and that will allow you to really serve and be there for others. But before you can open to the energy of love, you must learn to be fully present in your life. You must get yourself here.

This is why it's so important to be in your body, to understand the workings of your mind, to listen to and trust your feelings, and to be as conscious as you can be in your relationships, your work, in everything you do. As you become more committed to your healing journey, you'll discover that love is why you are here.

The door to love is through the heart. Only you can discover what's inside your heart. It means keeping your heart open, listening to and feeling for what's inside. You must trust what you feel. You must have the courage and compassion to experience your own pain and suffering. Stay with the process, and the energy will soon shift. The pain and constriction in your heart, caused by the past hurts that you and every other human being have suffered, will soften and give way to the love that is your real nature.

It's a lifelong journey, this opening of the heart. Yet it's the journey that promises the greatest happiness. Again and again, as you meet with disappointment and frustration, you'll want to close down, you'll want to withdraw, to disengage. Sometimes withdrawal is necessary, a time to regroup, to lick your wounds, to get clear. It's an opportunity to sort out what is and is not true for you.

If you're serious about your quest for wholeness, however, the call of the heart cannot be ignored for long. The happiest people are those whose hearts are fully open to life—the mystery, the wonder, the pain, the joy. There is no other way to freedom.

The Teaching of Jean Klein

All my teachers helped, in their different ways, to point me back to the beauty and love that was in me. Of them all, the one who pointed most directly—perhaps because there was no judgment, no criticism, nothing personal in his pointing—was Jean Klein. Tradition says that when the pupil is ready, the teacher appears. When Jean Klein came into my life, I was indeed ready for him.

He was in his seventies when I met him. He was a man of medium height, very slender, with a strong nose and a head of white hair that, while thin on top, was full and swept back like wings at the sides. An urbane, cultured European, he was a former medical doctor who, when he was in his forties, had become dissatisfied with the materialism in Europe and had gone to India in search of a more authentic way of being. As he was ready for a new outlook on life, he soon came across a man, a professor of Sanskrit, who became his teacher, his spiritual master. Within a few years he had come to a deep awakening within himself, and his life since that time has been given to sharing his understanding with others.

What attracted me to him—as it did so many other Westerners—was that he himself was from the West. He had been married, and had two grown children. He lived in Paris and loved art, music, and philosophy. He enjoyed good food and drank a glass of wine occasionally. He spoke our language (albeit with a thick accent!). He dressed like us and looked like us. We could relate to him.

His teaching was universal, but it had its roots in the Advaita Vedanta tradition, where Reality is held to be nondual, a term which means, literally, "not two." In the nondual approach, every "thing," every event—including our own human nature—is regarded as a manifestation of the one divine consciousness.

All reality is an expression of the play—or *lila*—of God, of Brahman, of the intelligence behind it all. God is not separate, not apart from us, in other words. In the nondual teaching, we're one with God. God is the ocean, and we're the waves on the ocean. The waves and the ocean are of the same substance. They only appear different. It's all one energy. The work of enlightenment is to realize this. It's to learn to rest in—and trust—our own divinity.

This perspective is the essence of Zen, of Taoism, of Sufism, and of the Gnostic, or mystical tradition in Christianity. It also happens to be the way modern quantum physics perceives reality. The physicist may not use the term "divine," but he does understand that, fundamentally, the only thing that is "real" is energy, and that all matter—all form and appearance—is but a manifestation of the one intrinsic, Absolute energy.

The more commonly held view of spiritual reality—the one that has traditionally appealed to the religious "masses"—is that God is separate from us. This is the dualistic perspective: there's "us," and then there's "God." In the dualistic paradigm, I believe in myself as a separate psychological identity, an "ego" or "self"—and I believe in God as an entity, or force, outside me.

The spiritual journey is therefore seen as a long and difficult struggle toward some hoped-for union with God. It's because of this feeling of distance from God that we so often feel unworthy and unloved. Moreover, because we take our personal "self" to be real, our frequent inner experience is one of anxiety, insecurity, and fear as we seek to survive in a competitive and hostile world.

Enlightenment, or liberation—which is the "goal" of the non-dual tradition—is to see through this illusion of separateness. It's to see, to directly experience, that the observing "I" or "self" we have taken ourselves to be has no reality in and of itself. The pervasive feeling of being an "I," a separate "me," is an illusion we maintain through belief, memory, thought, and projection.

As we start to get free of this sense of "me" and "mine" through letting go of the mental and emotional concepts that reinforce it, we open up to our true nature, which is awareness, or pure consciousness. At those times when we're abiding in pure awareness, there's a natural harmonization of energies. This harmony is experienced as the peace, joy, and creative energy that is the manifestation of our true Self.

We still have an ego, but it becomes more transparent. We live increasingly from our essential I, from transcendent being. The light and beauty of spirit, the source, shines through us. It's a very liberated, expanded feeling. The more established we are in this awareness, the less sense there is of ourselves as being a "somebody" experiencing something. It's a complete letting go of attachment to states and experiences of any kind. It's to live without any self-concept or self-image.

This is why it is said that he who knows, doesn't say, while he who says, doesn't know.

You're Beautiful as You Are

I was first introduced to this teaching and to Jean's work through a book of his, *The Ease Of Being*. As soon as I opened the book I knew I was reading the words of a master, a man who had a deep understanding of truth and who had realized that understanding in his own life. Not long after coming upon the book I heard he was giving a public dialogue, and I went to experience him in person.

At the time, I was a fairly seasoned truth-seeker, even a somewhat jaded one. I was getting burned out with my spiritual quest and was in need of some new inspiration. As a result of the inner work I'd done, both psychological and spiritual, I'd come to a certain acceptance of myself. The world was a lot less threatening to me. Yet, deep down, I felt there was something missing. There was an emptiness inside me. I tended to go back and forth between moments of great peace and contentment, and times of considerable restlessness and searching.

I also had the feeling that there was still something *wrong* with me that I had to correct, some core imbalance that I needed to root out and eradicate. It seemed like all the spiritual teachings I'd followed over the years had told me, in one way or another, "You've fallen from Grace and you need to be saved." "You're not good enough as you are, and you need to live differently." "The way you live is not the true way; you need to change it." The message I received was that if I wanted to "succeed" spiritually I needed to work harder, to meditate more, to be more disciplined in all my habits and actions.

During one of the first times I sat to talk with Jean, I told him about some of the problems I faced, and what I thought I needed to do in order to change my life so that I could move closer to finding the inner peace I was seeking.

After I finished speaking, he just looked at me. His eyes sparkled. "Don't change anything," he said. "You're beautiful as you are."

I sat in what was almost a stunned silence as I contemplated his words. This wasn't what I'd expected him to say. A part of me didn't want to believe him. I was so identified with myself as a "seeker" that if what he'd said was true—and at some level I knew it was—then what had I been doing all these years? If I truly was beautiful as I was, how could I justify continuing to pursue some ideal of enlightenment? His words took the wind out of my spiritual sails.

Jean went on to explain that it was in the immediate environment of my own body, mind, and senses—and my family, my friends, and my work—that I would discover my real nature, my true identity. I needed to really look into and question who I was and what was actually so in my life, not chase after a figment of my spiritual imagination.

The Path of Self-Inquiry

It was through my relationship with Jean that I started on the path of self-inquiry. Self-inquiry is essentially a more active form of meditation. It's asking yourself the basic philosophical questions in life, such as: "Who am I?" "What is the meaning of life?" "Why am I here?" and "What happens when I die?"

These are the questions that, as you go more deeply into them, gradually lead you toward genuine self-knowing. They enable you to use your mental powers of discrimination to pierce through the illusions and fantasies that prevent you from living an authentic life.

The value of self-inquiry is that it brings in the element of reason. It marries science with spirituality, knowledge with faith. It blends logic with intuition. You need both for wholeness. Right understanding clears the mind of false concepts and beliefs, opening the way for a deeper and more intuitive perception of reality. It orients your mind, points you in the direction of truth.

Right understanding helps you realize that happiness doesn't lie outside yourself in objects, people, things, circumstances, beliefs or ideals, because these are always changing. There can be no lasting happiness in something that is going to disappear, move on, or die. In this way, right understanding helps you give up grasping at things that are never going to produce the happiness you seek. It helps you get quiet and centered within, sensitive to something deeper in life, something timeless that is always here. Right understanding shifts your gaze from outside to back within, for it's inside you, in your heart—your spiritual nature—that what you're looking for resides.

It's also important to have an understanding of the experiences that happen to you along the way. Self-inquiry teaches you how to hold your experience, how to fit it into a conceptual framework that you can then work with and apply in your life (even though, eventually, you'll drop the conceptual framework). It gives you a working perspective, and without a perspective—a clear vantage point—it's all too easy to get lost or confused.

You end up going down paths that lead nowhere. For example, you may have a particularly profound or blissful experience and then, because it's so different than your normal state, you try to hold onto it, or recreate it. You develop an addiction to the experience and miss the whole point of spirituality, which is to let go of the attachment to every past experience, and be open to life, to being, in this moment now.

You may meet a spiritual teacher who has a certain power, and in his or her presence, you begin to grow. Because you associate growth with the teacher, you then get attached to the teacher. A teacher whose awakening is still immature, who still has too much ego in the way, encourages this kind of attachment because it supports his or her own insecurities, the need to be recognized and validated. It's very tempting to worship or idolize a strong teacher, and to regard him or her as the holder and giver of life, of power.

Sometimes it takes years, decades, to see through the error of this. Then you have to go through the pain of letting go of the outer teacher—the false God—and finding yourself in relationship to the true God within you. This is why in Zen it is said, "If you meet the Buddha on the road, kill him." Such a statement shocks us at first, because it sounds so sacrilegious. Yet there's great wisdom in it. The essence of Buddhist teaching is that the Buddha is in you. If you think he's outside, you're making a big mistake. So kill that illusion the moment it arises.

Going Deeper into Silence

It's mature understanding that enables you to see these traps and pitfalls, and frees you from being a victim of forces that often seem beyond your control. It's this same understanding that leads to spiritual insight, or enlightenment. Without it, you can meditate for years, and while you may find an element of peace and serenity in your meditation, living in the world and dealing with daily life will continue to be a problem.

Without an intuitive appreciation for the dynamic nature of life—its beauty, its wholeness, its divinely intelligent unfolding—meditation tends to become a cop-out. When meditation is used as an escape from the demands and responsibilities of daily life, it results in a drying-up of your creativity, rather than a blossoming of it. True enlightenment, remember, always brings you back into the world. It brings you more fully into everyday life, with all the joys, pleasures, problems, and challenges that everyday living entails.

The paradox of self-inquiry, of attaining a clear conceptual understanding of truth, is that eventually you come to the point where you realize that everything you "know," everything you've come up with in response to such questions as "Who am I?" is actually meaningless! You come to the realization that words, concepts, and beliefs only get in the way of genuine understanding.

You come to see that it's only in silence, the creative emptiness out of which thinking and speaking arise, that the perfume of life is to be found. To come to this knowing, this deep inner silence, you must exhaust all your mind's questions and concerns. You must deal with your mind, you must go through it in order to get beyond it. In true silence, or stillness, you begin to feel a quality of presence, of *beingness*, of deep harmony and order. It dawns on you that this presence, this feeling of unconditional awareness, or consciousness, is who and what you really are. You can give this awareness a name, but names—like any other concept—usually just get in the way.

As you learn to trust this silence, your seeking reaches its end. Your questions dissolve and become irrelevant. Thoughts come and go but they're not a problem, for they appear against the background of something much larger—the creative current of life itself, the beauty and fullness of *being*. You become one with being. Indeed, in those moments there's no "you" to speak of. There's only space, openness, and a boundless feeling of well-being, of joy.

The Short Path and the Long Path

Once you've discovered this quality of inner presence, then the challenge is to embody it, and to bring it into the everyday world of your work and your relationships. This is seldom an easy process. When you've begun to discover the source of spiritual peace within you, it's all too tempting to want to get lost there, to remain there.

The ordinary, everyday world, with all its potential for struggle, pain, and disappointment, can at times seem a very unappealing and depressing place. Yet come back to it you must, if you want to live your spirituality, if you want to be able to utilize what you know inwardly in a creative and meaningful way. Otherwise, your life will be out of balance.

Paul Brunton, the late writer and philosopher who did so much to introduce Westerners to the spiritual traditions of the East, speaks of this danger in the book, *Advanced Contemplation: The Peace Within You*. "They enter the region of the dark who are occupied solely with the finite," he says, quoting the *Iso Upanishad*, one of the Hindu scriptures, "But they fall into a region of still greater darkness who are occupied solely with the Infinite."

Brunton wisely emphasized the need for balance, for integrating the quest for spiritual fulfillment with a normal, active life in the world. He referred to Advaita Vedanta's non-dual teaching as the "Short" or "Direct" Path to truth. The more common dualistic tradition he called the "Long" or "Indirect" path. This is the slow, steadily progressing journey toward wholeness.

While he always spoke of the Short Path as the most direct way to truth, or realization, Brunton also took care to highlight the positive features of the Long Path. Among these are the disciplines and practices that make your body healthier, that bring your energies into more optimal alignment, and that center and ground your awareness in the here-and-now. The Long Path teaches of the necessity for learning to be more compassionate, more kind, and more conscious in the way you perform your work.

From the Short Path you learn that your real nature is God, or Self, and that your work is to let go of the false concepts that support the notion of being an ego, a separate "self." The direct path is a path of perception, of discrimination, of discernment. You're learning to see differently, to see the error of self-judgment, beliefs, assumptions, and all the other ways you reinforce the false sense of "self."

You're learning to see yourself instead as beautiful, whole, perfect as you are. You're learning to see yourself as already enlightened, rather than to regard yourself as an imperfect human being in need of change and self-improvement. It's accepting that there truly is nowhere to go, nothing to seek. That which you're looking for, you already are. It's within you—nearer to you, even, than your own breath.

Be Kind

Jean Klein, while primarily a Short Path teacher, always acknowledged the benefit of some of the Long Path techniques and practices. The yoga he taught, which I described in Chapter Four, is an example of this, as are some of the breathing exercises he would have his students do. Then, too, he'd sometimes (though not often enough for many of us!) give his students practical advice as to how to deal with certain problems.

For instance, a woman once spoke to him of the pain she was experiencing in her relationship with her lover. Her lover, who was not on any kind of a spiritual path at all, often treated her badly, to the point of being emotionally abusive, and she didn't know what to do about it.

"According to your teaching, I understand that there's really no 'me,' no 'person' to be hurt. But the fact is I feel hurt!" Her voice was pained as she spoke.

Jean smiled gently. "You're right," he said, "From the ultimate perspective, the person, the psychological entity who feels hurt and who suffers, doesn't exist. One day you'll realize this and you'll be free. In the meantime, from a practical standpoint, it's important that human beings be kind to one another. If someone is being unkind, it's better not to be around them."

I was quite moved by this interchange. I'd already begun to see that one of the pitfalls of the nondual, or Short Path, especially for someone to whom "spiritual awakening" was still such a cherished ideal, was that it tended to foster intellectual arrogance and emotional aloofness.

Da Free John, a contemporary American spiritual teacher, once called the Advaita tradition the "talking school" of enlightenment. Intellectually or philosophically-inclined individuals like myself could all too easily master the "rap," the teaching, and then begin to espouse it as if it were our own genuine inner experience, when in fact it was just another "head trip"—one more way of avoiding and denying the reality of feelings and emotions.

Listening to Jean counsel this woman reminded me that it was enormously valuable to understand the perspective he was teaching because it did, indeed, point to our true nature. Yet it was equally important—perhaps even more so—to learn to be a good and kind human being, no matter what one's "path," no matter what one's philosophical or cosmological view of life. In other words, it's not what you understand with your mind that matters, but the degree to which your heart is open. The mind has to come to clarity, but without a compassionate heart, the healing energy of love we seek cannot be felt or expressed.

The Relationship between Emotional and Spiritual Work

My own approach to spirituality, the one that I've shared with you throughout these pages, has been to combine the wisdom and understanding of the Short Path with the practical, "how-to-do-it-in-the-real-world" methods of the Long Path.

In this regard, I often think of the Buddha's Middle Way, or Middle Path. There have been teachers and *gurus* throughout history who have gained our attention through their vigorous declamations of truth, and their conviction that *their* particular way to God is better than or superior to everyone else's. The actual truth,

I've discovered, invariably lies somewhere in the middle, between the many extremes.

At the time I met Jean, I was just beginning to deal with this question of my "real" spiritual nature, versus my role, or function, as a man trying to make it in the world as a husband, father, and member of my community. I was looking for that balance point where the conflicts within me and in my life could resolve themselves into a more harmonious and unified whole.

When I read *The Ease Of Being* I was just completing an intensive year of transformational work with Stephano Sabetti. Under Stephano's guidance I'd been learning, with a group of others, what it meant to be grounded, to feel powerful in my body, to allow the feelings of fear, grief, and anger to have their way with me. I'd been learning how to release long-repressed emotional energy so that I could be more present in my life. I was beginning to let go of my attachment to analytical thinking and conceptual understanding, and get more into my feelings, into my actual bodily experience.

After a session of crying or raging with Stephano, when I was feeling spent, I'd often think of yoga and meditation, and this new perspective I was learning from Jean—his quiet, unassuming approach to truth—and wonder about the connection between the two kinds of work. What did emotional catharsis have to do with the subtle yoga movements that Jean taught, the yoga that was helping me become more sensitive in body and mind? What did it have to do with sitting in stillness and attuning to my real nature? What did it have to do with learning to shift my focus of attention from my personal "self" to the background, the global awareness that was behind it?

I mulled over these questions for quite a long time, and then one day I saw it: the emotional work was making me more available to meditation, to spiritual discernment. It was freeing up my energy, loosening my inner psychological contraction so that I could open up to other dimensions of awareness.

I remember asking Jean about this work and whether it was valuable in his view to learn to express one's anger, one's pain, to beat it out on a pillow if necessary. He replied that what was important was the acknowledgment of the feeling, the giving of space to it so that the energy was not repressed or denied.

He cautioned, however, that there must be awareness too, a witnessing of the feeling or emotion, otherwise the "I," the ego, would take over. It would clutch at this new-found ability to feel, emote, express itself, and in doing so would create yet another attachment.

How the Ego Gets in the Way

Understanding the ego's endless games was at the heart of Jean's teaching. It was the same message I'd heard from Krishnamurti, the man who had first opened my spiritual eye. It was what I'd learned from my study of Zen. It was the unifying thread that ran through all the wisdom traditions I'd examined.

The problem, the one thing in life that prevents us from awakening to our inner spiritual nature, is this "me," this ego that we've all spent so many years building and fortifying. "The less there is of I, the more there is of God," said Meister Eckhart. Or, as Jean put it, "Liberation consists in being free from the me."

When I met Jean I'd come to a point in my meditations where I'd begun to touch a state of bliss, a definite feeling of peace, of oneness with spirit. I'd learned how to let go of thought, to clear my mind, to be still in my body. I'd feel moments of wholeness and harmony during the day, and my spiritual "work" had become directed toward trying to have this feeling all the time, to bring it into every area of my life.

I wanted to believe that bliss was enlightenment, so I felt disappointed when I heard Jean say, "Enlightenment isn't a feeling, nor is it a state of bliss. All such states and sensations are objects which keep you bound, no matter how subtle and pleasant they are. They are delectations for the 'me,' sweets for the ego, that's all."

For a long time I resisted Jean's words. I'd spent my life searching for inner peace and now that I'd found it—so I believed—I wasn't about to willingly let it go. But in time I saw the truth in what he was saying. My own life began to show me how attached I'd become to the blissful state. The further I went in my meditation, the more conflict I experienced in my outer life. How real was my inner peace if it could be broken so easily by a family crisis, or my son coming in and disturbing me at the wrong time? I saw that the problem was not the bliss itself, but the *attachment* to it—the "me" jumping in and claiming it for itself.

Seeing all this, how my ego, my personal "I," still wanted to hold onto certain states, gave me a new sense of freedom. Gradually, I began to let go of my attachment. I learned to just allow whatever feelings and sensations were there, to simply be there. The result of this more flowing, non-attached approach to my meditation was that usually within a few minutes of sitting, all the contracted energy in my body/mind would dissolve, and the most delightful sensation of ease would begin to unfold.

The less I held onto this new feeling, I discovered—the less "me" there was in the picture—the more it would be there.

An Experience of Enlightenment

A few summers after I met Jean, I was at an eight-day retreat with him at Mount Madonna Center, in the Santa Cruz mountains in California. Jean had consistently spoken and written of the illusion of the personal self, and that enlightenment was seeing through the "me." It was seeing that the "me" didn't even really exist, that it was a fabrication held together by memory, belief, and conditioning. "Once the idea of being someone disappears, we find a peace which is ultimate reality," he would often say.

It was during this retreat that I began to contemplate the notion that my personal "I," my psychological center, might not be so real after all. I saw how so much of my spiritual journey had actually been a refining of my ego, so that while it looked as though I was more surrendered to the flow of things, in fact I was just more subtly and insidiously in control of myself. I saw the extent to which I was still caught in psychological conflict, and how it was this sense of "me" that I clung to that was the root cause of my suffering.

All of this became startlingly clear to me as I was strolling down to one of the afternoon dialogues. My "I," my ego-center, suddenly jumped out into my awareness and I saw, in an instant, the game I'd been playing. It was as if I was standing outside myself. I saw this "me" that I'd spent a whole lifetime cultivating, and I saw that it was a fiction. I'd been making up a story about myself and my life—especially around the notion of myself as a seeker of truth, and therefore someone special—for many, many years, and I'd believed it!

With this insight came a piercing sadness, a sense of loss. Now that I'd had a glimpse of the "me," this cherished image of myself that I'd invested so much energy in constructing, somehow I knew my relationship with it could never be quite the same. The sadness passed after half an hour or so, as spontaneously as it had appeared, and I became aware of a feeling of expansiveness and freedom.

During the dialogue, I told Jean about my experience. "Go home," he said, "See your life from an undivided mind, a choiceless mind free from selection. You'll do what has to be done, but you won't become the doer. Live completely in the absence of yourself, and you'll become a happy man."

All I'd ever wanted was to become a happy man. Wasn't the whole point of the spiritual journey to bring suffering to an end, so that we could all live happily with ourselves with each other?

After I returned to my normal life, that sense of "me," of ego, came back. It's one thing to taste enlightenment at a mountain retreat center; it's quite another to live with it in the everyday world, with all its demands around relationship, work, and economic survival.

For a little while at that retreat, however, there was no "me" at all. There was just the flow of awareness, that timeless sense of Being, our home-ground, as Jean liked to call it. In this awareness there was immensity, love, and a feeling of gratitude toward the man who had guided me to the understanding of all this.

The End of the Quest

The experience in the Santa Cruz mountains with Jean marked a turning point for me. Soon after it, I realized I was no longer a spiritual seeker in the way I'd been. For now I'd found what I sought. Now I knew the way Home, I knew the way back to that feeling of peace and well-being that is the source of all our experience, that is the ground of our very existence. I'd seen the small "I," my ego, my personality, for what it was, and I knew I was not that "I."

I was not the "person" I'd taken myself to be. I was not the beliefs and circumstances with which I'd identified myself. I was not my body, mind, or senses. They were expressions of me, but they were not the real me. My essence, my true identity, was that quality of openness and presence, of freedom and joy, I'd awakened to during the retreat.

At last I was beginning to release the attachment to my ego. Whether I ever attained some "final" state of enlightenment or not was now no longer an issue. If such a state of consciousness or being did exist, I knew it would only come about through Grace. There was no way "I" could get myself there. As Krishnamurti once said, in response to a questioner who asked what he could do to free himself from conflict, "There's nothing you can do. *You* are the problem."

Likewise, I could no longer escape the fact that "I" was the cause of my own internal suffering. My ego was all that stood between me and freedom. Whenever I felt myself feeling ill-at-ease, cut off from my spiritual source, it was because there was too much "me" in my life. The remedy, the cure, was to get myself quiet and still, and simply be present with all my energy and attention. Awareness itself would soon reveal the harmony that is at the heart of life, and in that harmony would be peace and contentment. It is *always* here, I came to realize. I just had to stop—that is, get myself out of the way by not "doing" anything—and it would unfold. This was the great discovery.

I think you'll find that your path will lead you to the same place. It will bring you to the intuitive realization that you are more than your body, mind, and circumstances—that your real nature is of God, of spirit. Once you've awakened to this, you'll have access to an inexhaustible well of creativity and joy, to an inner happiness that no one will be able to take from you.

No one will be able to take this happiness from you precisely because it *is* your nature. It's who and what you most fundamentally are. There'll come a day when even the changing events and circumstances of your life won't affect it. This happiness, the vitality inside you, will become a constant. It will always be here, the ever-present background music in the cosmic symphony that is your life.

Your spiritual mission is to tap into it.

Bringing It All Home

At one of the Mount Madonna dialogues, someone asked Jean what would happen if everyone in the world became enlightened. Jean looked at the questioner and was silent for a moment or two—the perfect picture of the wise old sage, pondering a serious question. Then suddenly he broke into a boyish grin and his eyes twinkled. "Why, there would only be dancing!" he said, in his thick French accent.

Looking back, I can see that I started my spiritual journey because I was looking for a way to live in the world, a way that would work, that would satisfy, that would feel right. I was looking to dance. All along, I was seeking to bring my spiritual understanding into daily life. Jean assisted me in doing that by pointing out the error of getting attached to bliss and other states, and by showing me, through the mirror of his own clarity, my real nature, the light that was in me.

All my teachers helped, in their own unique ways, to bring me back to myself. One of them, a therapist named Ernestine Ward, spent a year working on getting me into my body. Trained in energy work and body-oriented psychotherapy, Ernie saw the split between my mind, body, and spirit, and was relentless in her reminders to just be present with what I was experiencing.

"Forget walking in the hills or dissolving in meditation," she'd say, as she gently brought me back into the now moment. "Just stay in your body, stay with your feelings. This is where reality is. This is where spirit is. It's right here, right now. It's not out 'there'."

You'll find these things out too, if you haven't already done so. You too will discover that God is either "right here, right now," or is nowhere. It's absurd, when you reflect on it, to confine your experience of spirituality to certain favorite places, or certain special times. The work is to come back to the present, to this moment now, and feel the energy that's here. Through facing yourself each moment of the day, you discover how well your inner peace stands up. This means dealing not only with the problems and crises of daily living, but also the uneventfulness, the ordinariness, of it.

If you're concerned about the state of the world and are serious about seeing the conflict between peoples and nations healed, then you have to learn how to act in the marketplace with the same quality of equanimity you experience when you sit in a quiet place and meditate.

It's as you learn to be more fully present in every aspect of your life that true inner peace will start to become a reality for you. It comes in moments at first, this peace, and then those moments begin to increase, so that peace, rather than conflict, becomes more and more your natural state. And the key lies in getting yourself out of the way, in "living in the absence of yourself," as Jean put it to me.

This means learning to open up to spirit, that deeper energy we call God, or Buddha-nature, and trusting it. The more you open to it, the more you see the limits of your own mind and ego. You begin to live from your heart. You give yourself more and more to that energy, that current of love, so that increasingly it guides your entire life. When this starts to happen, you understand the significance of the scriptural phrase, "In Him we live, and move, and have our being."

When those moments of peace and clarity, of true expansiveness come, take note of them. This is very important. Feel the peace in your body. Consciously acknowledge the quality of spiritual presence, of harmonious energy, that's stirring within you. Don't dismiss that presence as something external to you, as simply a "peaceful moment." This is why real peace keeps eluding us. We've convinced ourselves that it's outside us, that it all depends upon some fortuitous combination of circumstances.

When the global feeling is there, really open up to it. Go into the stillness. Explore it. Accept that the sense of peace and stillness you're touching is, indeed, your real nature. Do this and it will help anchor the feeling in your body, in the depths of the being. Then you'll have it as an organic, cellular memory, and the state of enlightened awareness will be that much easier to find next time.

So often we think that the spiritual journey is going to lead us to some extraordinary place, to something very different than what we're experiencing now. Yet the great irony—the cosmic joke, you might say—is that the journey always, eventually, leads us back to ourselves, to the present moment, to the riches that are here. These inner riches are for you to discover. This is the spiritual treasure that awaits you, as you find out—and remember—who you are.

Let me close this final chapter with some words a friend passed on to me. I don't know who penned them, but they're a beautiful description of the spiritual journey.

> And yet who of you knew the full implications
> of what it meant to cry for wholeness?
> To know truth?
> And yet all of you knew it was unalterably your true path,
> and chose it willingly and surely, however blindly.
> So it is for humanity now,
> and those of you who can must sing the song of peace,
> and light the way home.

"This is something most marvelous if you can come upon it. I can go into it, but the description is not the described. It's for you to learn all this by looking at yourself—no book, no teacher can teach you about this. Don't depend on anyone, don't join spiritual organizations; one has to learn all this out of oneself. And there the mind will discover things that are incredible. But for that, there must be no fragmentation and therefore immense stability, swiftness, mobility. To such a mind there is no time and therefore living has quite a different meaning."

Conclusion

Above is the full statement behind the Krishnamurti quote with which I began this book. It comes from the last page of the slim, elegant volume called *Meditations*, a book which contains the essence of Krishnamurti's teaching around meditation. It is a beautiful book, the kind you can let fall open at any page, and discover a gem—a few words, a paragraph—that in itself speaks reams about the art and mystery of living.

It may seem strange to end a book about healing and spirituality with a quote that states very clearly that such things can't be learned from a book! Yet this is the way of the spiritual journey: it is full of paradox. We seek the truth, we seek answers to our questions, we seek solutions to our problems through books, teachers, organizations, and for a while it seems as though they do help us.

Yet, as I've said elsewhere in these pages, the truest teachers and the truest books always, in the end, point you back to yourself. They point you back to the silence and spaciousness within you, to your own wisdom and knowing. You may remember the book or teacher with gratitude and affection, but increasingly you come to the place where you now no longer need either. You've found the energy within you. You've found your *Self*. You're free.

This book has come out of my own journey, which includes the workshops that I love to share with others. The workshop experience itself is special, as I intimated in the Introduction, because it gives people a chance to actually feel the spiritual energy that is at the heart of life. It gives them an opportunity to have a direct experience of who they really are.

By the end of a workshop, the energy is always strongly evident in the room. Our bodies have settled, our minds have quieted, we're together in silence. Our hearts are open, our attention is here. There's a feeling of love and unity, of ease and naturalness between us all. We're simply and unconditionally present with each other.

For a few people in the room, the workshop has been like an emotional roller-coaster. They've gone through many different spaces, and have experienced feelings coming alive within them that they may not have felt in a long time. For the majority, however, it's been a deepening, expanding experience. They feel more fully themselves than they did at the beginning of the workshop. For some, this feeling of being totally integrated, centered in body, mind, and spirit, is an entirely new feeling—so new that it feels like a rebirth.

We finish the workshop sitting—usually on cushions—in a circle. We join hands, left palm up to receive the current of energy from the person on our left, right palm down to allow it to flow easily and effortlessly to the person on our right. There's a wonderful resonance between us, a powerful sense of being joined, connected at the heart.

After any final sharing (and there's never a lot that needs to be said by this stage; we're so nourished by the silence that words become superfluous), I often conclude by explaining how people greet—and say goodbye—to each other in India. I tell them how they join their hands in salute and say, "*Namaste.*"

The short meaning of the word is, simply, "I salute the God in you," but there's a longer meaning, one which I learned from Ram Dass, in his book, *Grist for the Mill.* It goes like this:

I honor the place in you where the entire universe resides, I honor the place in you of love, of light, of truth, of peace. I honor the place within you where if you are in that place in you and I am in that place in me, there is only one of us.

After I've shared this with the group, I raise my palms together in front of me, smile, and say, "*Namaste.*"

There's a ripple in the room. Just about everyone breaks into a spontaneous smile themselves. Even those who have never done any form of yoga and who know nothing about Eastern ways, respond by bringing their hands together simultaneously, and saying in unison, "*Namaste.*"

Then there's silence again, stillness. At this point there's so much love, so much good feeling in the room, that nobody moves. The workshop is over and yet no one wants to go. Who could leave this? The energy is very, very strong, a tangible current of peace and well-being moving through each of us, moving throughout the room.

During the workshop we've been touched and healed by this energy in various ways, and now we're literally bathed in it, nurtured by it. It has given each of us what we need, brought each of us back Home, reminding us of what is real, of what truly matters in life. Some of us, inevitably, get this more fully, more deeply than others, depending on where we are on our path and how much conflict we're dealing with, how far we've drifted, strayed from the source. But in this moment, at least, there's only love in the room. There is only Oneness.

After a few minutes, I make a move and everyone else, reluctantly, begins to stir. Soon, everybody is standing, saying their farewells to each other. Many of us hug, some exchange addresses, promises to get together again soon for more of this wonderful, heartfelt sharing. People gather their things and begin to leave.

We leave to go out into the world again, into a world that is sorely in need of this conscious, healing way of relating. It's not going to happen right away, but if enough of us keep honoring the truth in our own hearts and souls, eventually enough of humanity will sit up and take notice.

We'll all start to feel our connection to each other. We'll have more compassion for both our own pain and aloneness, and for the distress and suffering of others. We'll begin to tap the source of love itself, the love that is bigger than any of our racial, ethnic, religious, social, and political differences. The love that comes from that ultimate energy we call God, the source. The love that is the ground of our being, that is our true nature.

So now the real work begins.

Remember... Be still, look, listen, breathe. Feel the energy that's here. Discover the beauty and power of the present. It will change your life.

Index

209; becoming one with, 265; and body, 20; feeling of, 89; revealed in meditation, 85; as true identity, 52, 231

Beliefs: changing nature of, 50-51; and ego identity, 161-163; releasing through meditation, 83, 85, 91, 96; seeing limitation of, 105, 182

Bhagavad Gita, 189

Bible, 50, 223

Bioenergetics, 28

Blame, letting go of 137-140, 146

Bliss: attachment to, 90-91, 263; and enlightenment, 269-270; following your, 194-195

Body: affects mind, 33; and being present, 79, 163; centering exercise for, 23-25; awareness based in, 20; and meditation, 86-88; as mirror/metaphor, 22; therapies for, 24-25; Tibetan text on, 22

Boredom, 78

Boundaries: in relationships, 135-136, 141, 153; rigid vs. flexible, 79

Bradshaw, John, 135, 205

Brahman, 49, 259

Breathing, 13-17; chronic tension and, 15; as conscious exercise, 16-17; into feelings and emotions, 66-68; foundational spiritual practice, 14; and meditation, 86, 88; and releasing fear, 237-239

Brunton, Paul, 265

Buddha, 263; on power of thought, 42; on impermanence, 75

Buddha-nature, 11, 45, 49, 99, 109, 157, 201, 231, 274

Buddhism, and two aspects of enlightenment, 143

Burn-out, 160, 171

C

Campbell, Joseph, 194

Castaneda, Carlos, 6, 51. *See also* Don Juan

Children: and break-up of relationship, 149; conscious raising of, 140-141; dealing with conflict in; 101; and fathers; 125; innocence of, 69; and movement, 34; teaching responsibility to, 159-160, 173, 214-215

Chiropractic, 24, 28, 235-236

Choice: and commitment, 253-256; fear of making, 173-174; getting clear about, 174-178; making right, 250-253; power of, 46, 247-248; and responsibility, 243

Christ-consciousness, 49

Clarity: attaining, xviii, 48-49, 52-53, 177-184; becoming established in, 43-44; and freedom from addiction, 120; and Law of Attraction, 181; and meditation, 84-86

Co-creation, 100

Commitment: preceded by choice, 253-255; to spiritual awakening, 11

Communication, exercise for, 150-152

Compassion, 2, 280; as attribute of enlightenment, 143, 267; and freedom, 163

Compromise: as threat to well-being, 188; as trade-off, 176

Conflict: art of defusing, 103-105; caused by resistance, 97; creating out of, 98-99; inherent in mind, 162; learning from, 100-101, resolving in meditation, 137-139

Consciousness, as true nature, 53

Control, surrender and, 7-8
Course In Miracles, 106, 140, 163
Creating, 206; as life credo, 182-
183; out of conflict vs. wholeness, 98-100
Crisis: as wake-up call, xiii, 167-
169, and facing mortality, 235

D

Da Free, John, 267
Daily routine, 206-207
Decisions, making, 195
Demons, xv
Denial: moving out of, 105, 144-
145, 177; of problems, 161
Desire: influence of mind on, 196;
as innate human urge, 177; own-
ing and accepting, 104-105, 178
Dharma, 189
Diet: eating for energy, 35-40,
206-207; and emotional well-
being, 38-40; nutritional supple-
ments, 38; yogis and, 39
Discipline, and heightened aware-
ness, 70. *See also* Self-discipline
Disease. See Illness
Dishonesty, 254
Don Juan: on dropping personal
history, 51; on path with heart, 6
Drugs, 111-112, 167
Dualistic perspective, 260, 265
Durckheim, Karlfried Graf, 20, 22,
200, 208-209
Dying: facing death, 233-238; fear
of, xiii, 168; to moment, 231,
232; real self doesn't die, xviii-xix
Dzogchen, 89

E

Eckhart, Meister, 269
Ego, 20; addiction to, 114;
attempts to dissolve, 7; and

attachment, xv, 269-270; as
cause of relationship conflict,
122, 131, 144, 164; and choice,
175, 252-253; and conflict, xviii,
65, 163; and denial, 161; dissolves in love, 192; emphasis on
in West, 99; expanding beyond,
62; facing up to, 200; fall prey
to, 244; freedom from, 86, 93,
176, 225, 239, 255, 266, 270-
272; and "hard" eyes, 88; illusion of, 69, 175-176, 260,
270-272; as personal history, 50-
52, 232; rising above, 62 108-
109; transparency of, 9, 260
Einstein, Albert, 92, 166
Emotional baggage, 83, 149, 161
Emotional wounds, healing of,
134-145, 148-149
Emotions: diet and, 38-40; as
energy, 66; and healing from
within, 121-122, 228; natural
expression of, 231; relationship
between body and, 33-34; and
spiritual work, 267-269
Endarkenment, 229
Energy: art of "holding," 31;
becomes harmonious in meditation, 95; becoming sensitive to,
61-63; breathing into, 66; dysfunctional patterns of, 66; non-
linear, 178; releasing contracted,
64-65; working directly with, 4-
6. *See also* Spiritual energy
Enlightenment, 236; best diet for,
39; bringing into daily life, 29,
200-202, 264; difficulty of
describing, 5-6; experience and
definition of, xiv-xvi, 269-273; as
freedom from illusion, 119, 260;
"head trip," 267; *kensho*, 228;
lightening up, 229; and money,

212; problems don't go away, 158; quest for, 169-172, 174-175; *satori*, 201, 228; and self-acceptance, 101; as wisdom and compassion, 143; work of, 259

Entropy, 159

Exercise, two types needed, 32, 206

F

Fear: begins to drop away, xviii; breathing through, 237-239; as paralysis, 28. *See also* Dying

Feelings: breathing into, 60-61; come in waves, 67-68; importance of in healing, 60, 273; learning language of, 129-130; opening to, 55-57, 268-269; trusting, 59;

Feminine energy: and *animus*, 124; bringing into balance, 124-125, 131-132; healing power of, 127-129; nature of, 123-124; opening to, 129-130; qualities of, 4

Flow: of awareness, 271; going with, 98

Forgiveness, 133; healing power of, 139-140; letting go of blame, 137; and self-acceptance, 107

Freedom: authentic, 54; deep desire for, 157-158; living in, 238

Friendship, 149

Future, getting in perspective, 73-76, 239

G

Gifts, distinguishing between talents and, 192-194

Global awareness, 253, 268

Goals: alignment with purpose, 178, 180; defining spiritual, 169-170; and patriarchal system, 126; provide a focus, 166; and relishing the journey, 74

Goddess movement, 127

Goodchild, Chloe, 156

Grace, xiii, 11, 99, 218, 272; and will, 8

Grateful Dead, 184

Gratitude, 217, 231; exercise for, 225; healing gift of, 223-226; lesson in, 218; and abundance, 218-219

Grief, 56-57, 68, 142, 146, 228, 231

Grounding: exercise for, 23-24, 98; importance of, 58, 67, 90

Guilt, 128-129

Gurdjieff, G. I., 23-24

Gurus. See Teachers

H

Hanna, Thomas, 20, 27

Hara, 24

Healing: as awakening to true identity, 52; as process of moving energy, 27-29; split between spirit and world, 162, 203, 216; as spiritual journey, 191-192

Heart: healing of, 143-144; living from, 274; opening, 258; path of, 142-144; speaks, 154

Herrigel, Eugen, xiv

Hesse, Herman, xiv, 168

Higher power, 99, 115-116

Hoffman, Bob: on healing anger and resentment, 145; *No One Is To Blame*, 138

Holy Spirit, 11

Homeopathy, 143

Honesty, need for with self, 170-171, 174, 182

233, 258; knows what to do,
195-197, something felt, 194-
195, 197; as source of inspiration
and focus, 190; taking time for,
191-192; and true purpose, 187

Perception, dictates reality, 221-223

Perspective, learning to shift, 53-54

Potential, fulfilling, 199

Prayer, 94-95, 218-219, 225

Presence, can be felt, 76-77

Present, living in, 73-80

Problems: mind creates, 162-163; not running from, 160-162; secret of dealing with, 163-164; solving through meditation, 84-86, 92-93; an unattended situation, 158-159; worry about them less, xviii, 239

Projection, 106

Psychoanalysis, 20

Psychotherapy, 157, 165; body-oriented approach, 28, 273; main contribution of, 61; transpersonal approach, 136; value and limitations, 135

Purpose: discovering true, 178-185, 187; clarity of, xvi

Q

Quantum physics, 27, 260

Question, leads to answer, 184, 240-241

R

Radix, 28

Ramakrishna, 52

Ram Dass, 200, 278

Reality: created by thoughts, 42; things moving, 27

Reichian work, 28

Rejection: facing pain of, 141-142, 153

Relationships: communicating truth in, 150-153; desire to heal, 136-137; ego destroys, 144; finding harmony in, 146-148, 230; genuine meeting, 154-155; great lesson in, 164; an inside job, 150, 152-153; problems in, 160; releasing blame, 137-140; and spiritual intimacy, 122; as spiritual process, 155-156; as teacher, 133, 155; unconscious patterns in, 148-150

Remen, Rachel Naomi, on the heart and healing, 144

Resentment, working through, 221-223

Resistance, and conflict, 97, 101-104

Risk, 251-252, 255

Rolfing, 25

Rumi, 59, 61, 240

S

Sabetti, Stephano: on importance of movement, 28-29; personal work with, 58-60, 66, 268

St. Francis, xv

St. Paul, 50

Satchitananda, xvi

Schiffmann, Erich, 232, 246-248

Self-acceptance, xix, 101-109; the first enlightenment, 101; the great peacemaker, 10-11, 108

Self-concept, 217, 234; letting go of need for, 51-53, 230, 261

Self-discipline, 202-205

Self-esteem, 135; in children, 160; not tied to circumstances, 158

Self-inquiry, 262-264

Self-knowing: and being present, 79-80; path to, 3

Self-realization, 184

Self-sabotage, 160

Self-will, 164. *See also* Ego

Separateness: as fundamental spiritual dilemma, 114-115; illusion of, 260. *See also* Enlightenment

Sex, as spiritual union, 122
Shadow, 205; accepting, 182; tendency to avoid, 6
Shah, Idries, 4
Shakespeare, W., 248, 252
Shiva, 29
Short Path, 265-267
Silence, going deeper into, 264-265; power of, 241
Sinclair clan, 209-210
Sobriety, promise of, 119-120
Socrates, 3
Somatic experience, 20
Soul: dark night of, 67-68; voice of 255
Spirit: beautiful quality of, 64-65; and creative inspiration, 190; energy is real, xx; healing power of, 121-122, 202; as real nature, 257, 272
Spiritual community, 122
Spiritual emergency, 90
Spiritual energy: attuning to, xvi, 180, 278; as current of well-being, xviii, 279; fears fall away, xviii; as presence, xiii, 274; a quickening, 5; source of everything, xix. See also Energy
Spirituality: addictions and, 114-116; as avoidance of feeling, 143; and conflict with material, 174; defining, 169-170; direct experience of, xiv; hunger for, 128; integration in daily life, xiv, 174, 209, 273-274
Spiritual quest, end of, 271-274
Spiritual well-being, as priority, 174-176
Stillness: tuning in to, 247, 268, 274; yoga as means to, 30-31
Strength, need for, 78-79
Success: breeds success, 223; and *dharma*, 189, resenting vs. wel-

coming, 181-182; winner's attitude, 42-43
Suffering: and attachment to past and future, 74-76; caused by ego, 272; and conflicting wants and desires, 166; getting free of images that cause, 61-63; healed by love, 268; negative thinking and, 43; a powerful teacher, 9
Sufis: and asking the right question, 184; and dealing with problems, 158
Surrender, 2; true meaning of, 7, 100-101
Suzuki, D.T., definition of enlightenment, xiv-xv
Suzuki Roshi, on beginner's mind, 83

T

Talents, distinguishing between gifts and, 192-194
Tantra, 29
Tao Te Ching: on dissolving hardness, 130; Master's secret, 128; no fight, no blame, 139; on suppleness, 34; *yin* and *yang* energies, 123-124
Teachers, xiv, 267; attachment to, 263; enlightened qualities of, 76-77, 277-278; limitation of, 10, 129; trusting, 245-246
Tears, melt hardness, 56-57, 59
Technology, advantages and limitations, 126
Tension: in body, 25; facial, 58-59; negative thinking and, 33; positive thinking and, 46; releasing through breathing, 14-15
Thinking: error of being identified with, 50; freedom from psychological, 54, 232; as instrument of awareness, 52, 232; letting go of

On the following pages you will find listed, with their current prices, some of the books now available on related subjects. Your book dealer stocks most of these and will stock new titles in the Llewellyn series as they become available. We urge your patronage.

TO GET A FREE CATALOG

You are invited to write for our bi-monthly news magazine/catalog, *Llewellyn's New Worlds of Mind and Spirit*. A sample copy is free, and it will continue coming to you at no cost as long as you are an active mail customer. Or you may subscribe for just $10 in the United States and Canada ($20 overseas, first class mail). Many bookstores also have *New Worlds* available to their customers. Ask for it.

In *New Worlds* you will find news and features about new books, tapes and services; announcements of meetings and seminars; helpful articles; author interviews and much more. Write to:

Llewellyn's New Worlds of Mind and Spirit
P.O. Box 64383-K244, St. Paul, MN 55164-0383, U.S.A.

TO ORDER BOOKS AND TAPES

If your book store does not carry the titles described on the following pages, you may order them directly from Llewellyn by sending the full price in U.S. funds, plus postage and handling (see below).

Credit card orders: VISA, MasterCard, American Express are accepted. Call us toll-free within the United States and Canada at 1-800-THE-MOON.

Special Group Discount: Because there is a great deal of interest in group discussion and study of the subject matter of this book, we offer a 20% quantity discount to group leaders or agents. Our Special Quantity Price for a minimum order of five copies of *The Ultimate Cure* is $59.80 cash-with-order. Include postage and handling charges noted below.

Postage and Handling: Include $4 postage and handling for orders $15 and under; $5 for orders *over* $15. There are no postage and handling charges for orders over $100. Postage and handling rates are subject to change. We ship UPS whenever possible within the continental United States; delivery is guaranteed. Please provide your street address as UPS does not deliver to P.O. boxes. Orders shipped to Alaska, Hawaii, Canada, Mexico and Puerto Rico will be sent via first class mail. Allow 4-6 weeks for delivery. **International orders:** Airmail – add retail price of each book and $5 for each non-book item (audiotapes, etc.); Surface mail – add $1 per item.

Minnesota residents add 7% sales tax.
Mail orders to:
Llewellyn Worldwide, P.O. Box 64383-K244, St. Paul, MN 55164-0383, U.S.A.
For customer service, call (612) 291-1970.

A CHAKRA & KUNDALINI WORKBOOK
Psycho-Spiritual Techniques for Health, Rejuvenation, Psychic Powers and Spiritual Realization
by Dr. Jonn Mumford (Swami Anandakapila Saraswati)

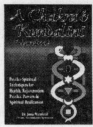

Spend just a few minutes each day on the remarkable psycho-physiological techniques in this book and you will quickly build a solid experience of drugless inner relaxation that will lead towards better health, a longer life, and greater control over your personal destiny. Furthermore, you will lay a firm foundation for the subsequent chapters leading to the attainment of super-normal powers (i.e., photographic memory, self-anesthesia and mental calculations), an enriched Inner Life, and ultimate transcendence. Learn techniques to use for burnout, mild to moderate depression, insomnia, general anxiety and panic attacks, and reduction of mild to moderate hypertension. Experience sex for consciousness expansion, ESP development, and positive thinking. The text is supplemented with tables and illustrations to bridge the distance from information to personal understanding. In addition, the author has added a simple outline of a 12-week practice schedule referenced directly back to the first nine chapters.

A Chakra & Kundalini Workbook is one of the clearest, most approachable books on Yoga there is. Tailored for the Western mind, this is a practical system of personal training suited for anyone in today's active and complex world.

1-56718-473-1, 296 pgs., 7 x 10, 8 color plates, softcover   **$16.95**

THE ART OF SPIRITUAL HEALING
by Keith Sherwood

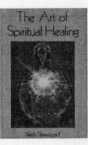

Each of you has the potential to be a healer; to heal yourself and to become a channel for healing others. Healing energy is always flowing through you. Learn how to recognize and tap this incredible energy source. You do not need to be a victim of disease or poor health. Rid yourself of negativity and become a channel for positive healing.

Become acquainted with your three auras and learn how to recognize problems and heal them on a higher level before they become manifested in the physical body as disease.

Special techniques make this book a "breakthrough" to healing power, but you are also given a concise, easy-to-follow regimen of good health to follow in order to maintain a superior state of being. This is a practical guide to healing.

0-87542-720-0, 224 pgs., 5 1/4 x 8, illus., softcover   **$7.95**

SECRETS OF A NATURAL MENOPAUSE
A Positive, Drug-Free Approach
by Edna Copeland Ryneveld

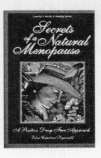

Negotiate your menopause without losing your health, your sanity, or your integrity! *Secrets for a Natural Menopause* provides you with simple, natural treatments-using herbs, vitamins and minerals, foods, homeopathy, yoga, and meditation-that are safer (and cheaper) than estrogen replacement therapy.

Simply turn to the chapter describing the treatment you're interested in and look up any symptom from arthritis, depression, and hair loss to osteoporosis and varicose veins—you'll find time-honored as well as modern methods of preventing or alleviating menopausal symptoms that *work,* all described in plain, friendly language you won't need a medical dictionary to understand.

For years, allopathic medicine has treated menopause as a disease brought on by a deficiency of hormones instead of a perfectly natural transition. *Secrets for a Natural Menopause* will help you discover what's best for *your* body and empower you to take control of your own health and well-being.

ISBN: 1-56718-596-7, 6 x 9, 224 pp., illus. $12.95

YOGA FOR EVERY ATHLETE
Secrets of an Olympic Coach
by Aladar Kogler, Ph.D.

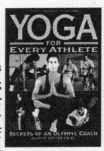

Whether you train for competition or participate in a sport for the pure pleasure of it, here is a holistic training approach that unifies body and mind through yoga for amazing results. The yoga exercises in this book not only provide a greater sense of well being and deeper unity of body, mind and spirit, they also increase your body's abil-ity to rejuvenate itself for overall fitness. Use the yoga asanas for warm-up, cool-down, regeneration, compensation of muscle dysbalances, prevention of injuries, stimulation of internal organs, or for increasing your capacity for hard training. You will experience the remarkable benefits of yoga that come from knowing yourself and knowing that you have the ability to control your autonomic, unconscious functions as you raise your mental and physical performance to new heights. Yoga is also the most effective means for accomplishing the daily practice of concentration. Yoga training plans are outlined for 27 different sports.

ISBN: 1-56718-387-5, 6 x 9, 320 pp., softbound $16.95